Salad Menu

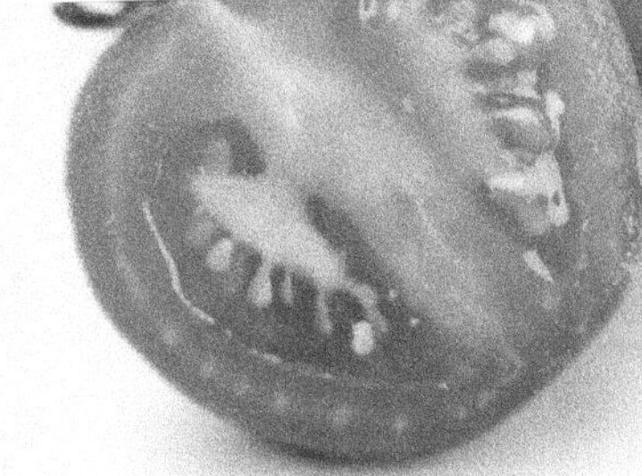

Introduction

Chapter 1: Leafy Greens and Cruciferous Delights

Salad *Menu*

Chapter 2: Protein-Packed Power Salads

Salad Menu

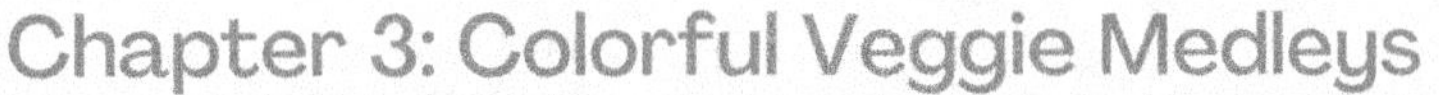

Chapter 3: Colorful Veggie Medleys

Salad Menu

Chapter 4: Nutty and Fruity Creations

Salad *Menu*

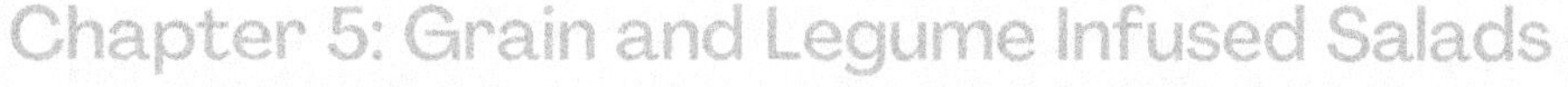

Chapter 5: Grain and Legume Infused Salads

Salad *Menu*

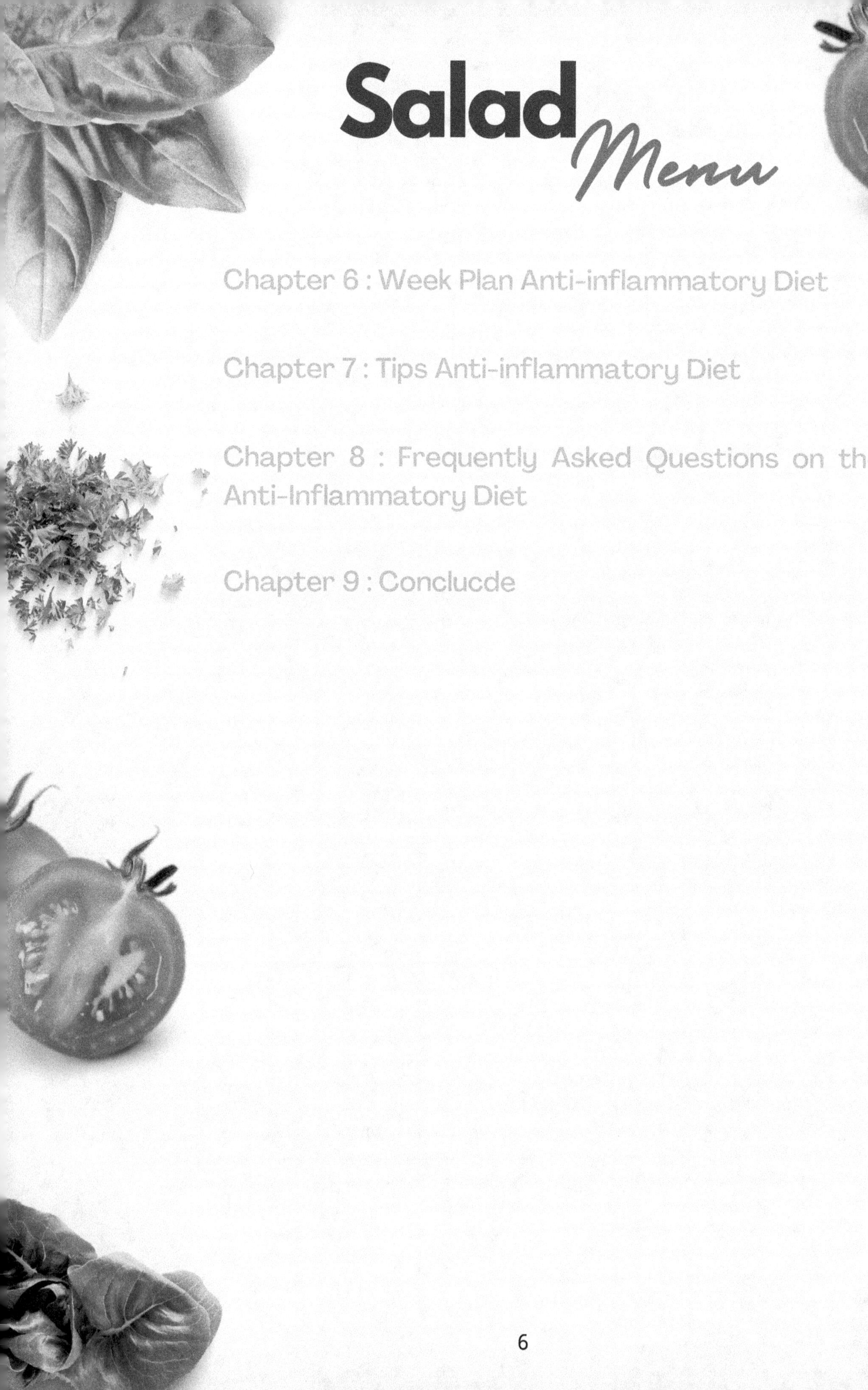

Introduction

Inflammation is a natural process that helps our bodies heal from injuries and fight off infections. However, chronic inflammation, when the immune system remains active for prolonged periods, can contribute to various health problems, including arthritis, heart disease, and diabetes. Diet plays a crucial role in managing inflammation, and one of the most effective ways to incorporate anti-inflammatory foods into your daily routine is through salads.

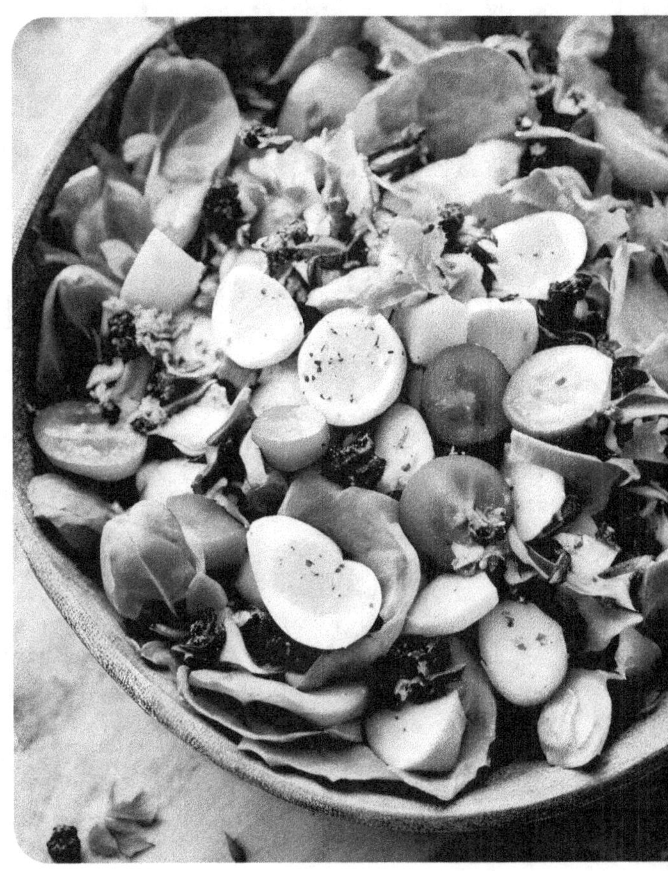

Salads offer a versatile and delicious way to combine a variety of nutrient-dense ingredients that combat inflammation. This cookbook is dedicated to providing you with an array of recipes that are not only delicious but also packed with anti-inflammatory benefits. From leafy greens and cruciferous vegetables to protein-packed ingredients and vibrant fruits, these salads will become a staple in your diet, promoting better health and well-being.

In this introduction, we will explore the science behind inflammation and how certain foods can help manage it. You'll learn about key anti-inflammatory ingredients, tips for preparing and storing salads, and how to customize these recipes to suit your taste and health needs. Let's embark on this journey to discover the healing power of food and how these simple, yet powerful, salads can make a difference in your life.

Understanding Inflammation and Diet

Inflammation is the body's response to harmful stimuli, such as pathogens, damaged cells, or toxic compounds. While acute inflammation is a protective mechanism, chronic inflammation can lead to various diseases. Diet plays a significant role in either exacerbating or alleviating inflammation. Consuming a diet rich in anti-inflammatory foods can help reduce chronic inflammation and improve overall health

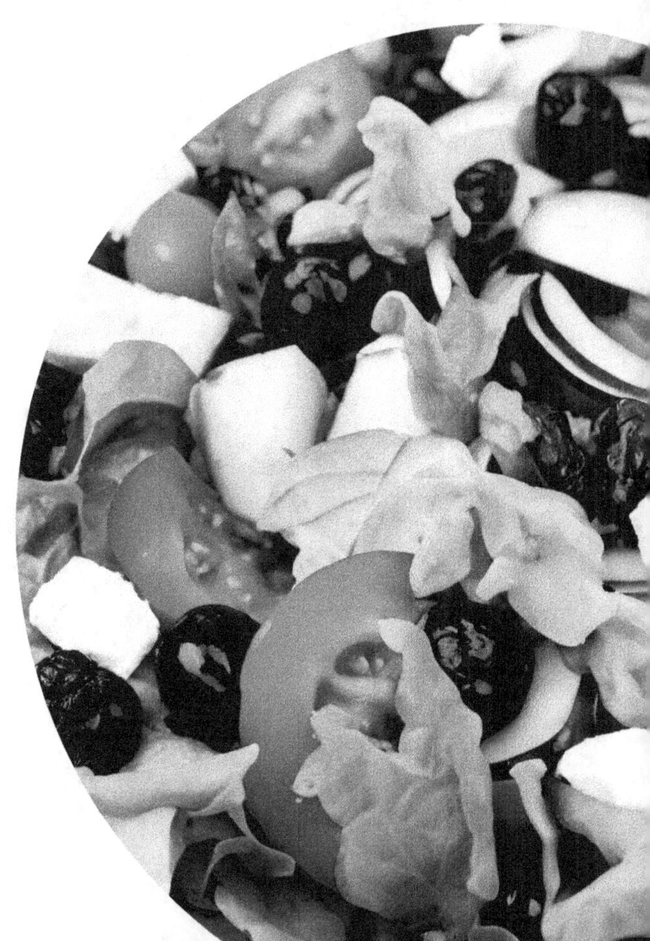

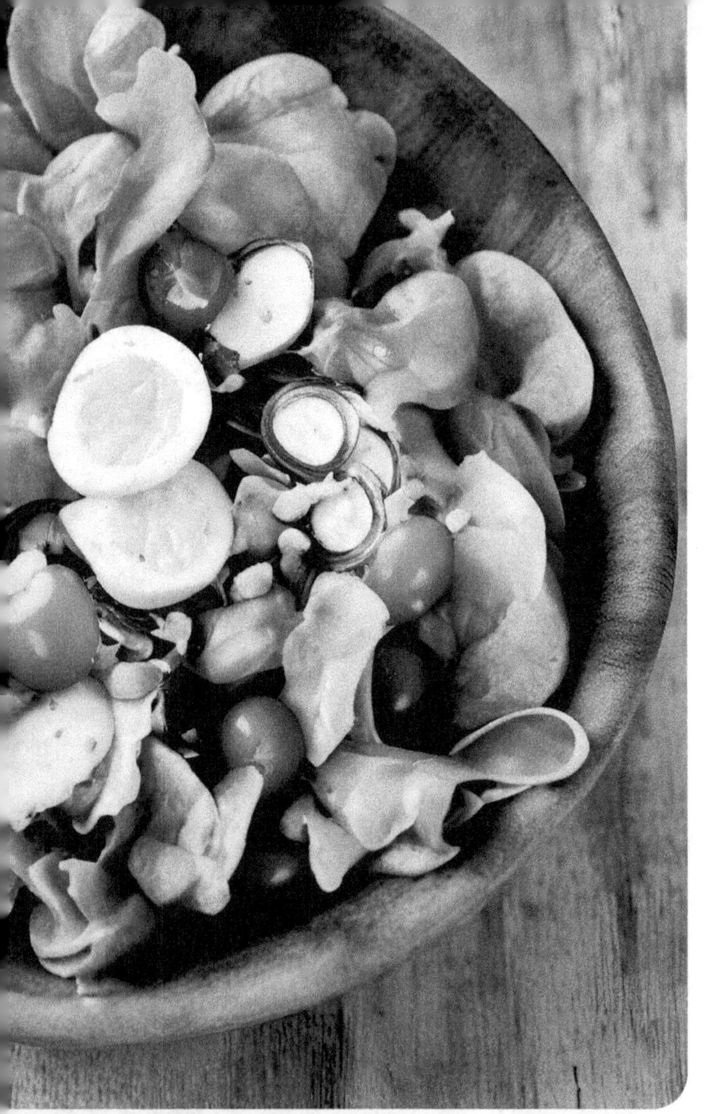

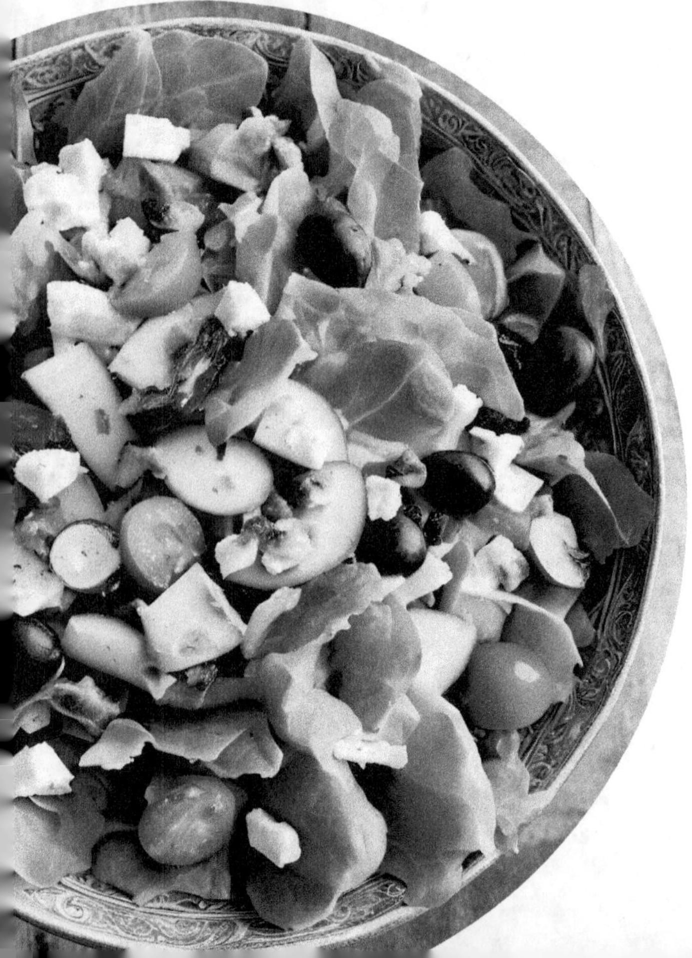

Benefits of Anti-Inflammatory Salads

Salads are an excellent vehicle for anti-inflammatory foods because they allow you to combine multiple ingredients that work synergistically to combat inflammation. They are also easy to prepare, versatile, and can be customized to fit any dietary preference or restriction. Additionally, salads are naturally rich in fiber, vitamins, minerals, and antioxidants, all of which contribute to reducing inflammation and promoting good health.

Key Ingredients for Inflammation Reduction

Certain foods are known for their anti-inflammatory properties. Leafy greens like kale and spinach, cruciferous vegetables such as broccoli and cauliflower, and berries like blueberries and strawberries are all powerful anti-inflammatory ingredients. Healthy fats from avocados, nuts, and seeds, along with lean proteins and whole grains, further enhance the anti-inflammatory benefits of these salads.

Tips for Preparing and Storing Salads

To make the most of your anti-inflammatory salads, it's essential to prepare and store them properly. Freshness is key, so always choose the highest quality ingredients available. Wash and dry your greens thoroughly to prevent wilting. Store dressings separately from the salad until ready to eat to keep everything crisp. Mason jars are excellent for storing salads, as they keep ingredients fresh and allow for easy transport.

By incorporating these tips and understanding the principles of an anti-inflammatory diet, you are well on your way to enjoying delicious, health-promoting salads. Now, let's dive into the first chapter and explore a range of leafy greens and cruciferous delights that will become staples in your anti-inflammatory arsenal.

 **Preparation: 15 minutes**

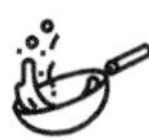 **Cook Time: 0 minutes**

 **Total Time: 15 minutes**

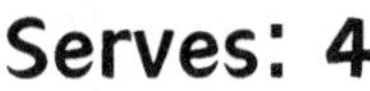 **Serves: 4**

1 bunch kale, stems removed and leaves chopped
- 1 avocado, diced
- 1/4 cup tahini
- 2 tablespoons lemon juice
- 2 tablespoons water
- 1 garlic clove, minced
- 1 teaspoon honey
- 1/4 teaspoon salt
- 1/4 teaspoon black pepper

1. Kale and Avocado Salad with Lemon-Tahini Dressing

1. In a large bowl, combine the chopped kale and diced avocado.

2. In a small bowl, whisk together the tahini, lemon juice, water, garlic, honey, salt, and pepper until well combined.

3. Pour the lemon-tahini dressing over the kale and avocado and toss to coat.

4. Serve immediately.

Nutrition Facts: Calories 220 | Total Fat 16g | Saturated Fat 2g | Cholesterol 0mg | Sodium 260mg | Total Carbohydrates 16g | Dietary Fiber 6g | Total Sugars 4g | Protein 6g

This salad is a great anti-inflammatory option, featuring nutrient-dense kale and heart-healthy avocado, all dressed in a creamy lemon-tahini dressing.

 **Preparation: 10 minutes**

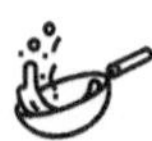 **Cook Time: 0 minutes**

 **Total Time: 10 minutes**

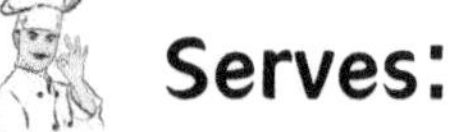 **Serves: 4**

5 oz baby spinach
- 1 cup fresh strawberries, sliced
- 1/4 cup sliced almonds
- 2 tablespoons white wine vinegar
- 1 tablespoon honey
- 1 tablespoon Dijon mustard
- 2 tablespoons olive oil
- 1 tablespoon poppy seeds
- 1/4 teaspoon salt
- 1/4 teaspoon black pepper

2. Spinach and Strawberry Salad with Poppy Seed Vinaigrette

1. In a large salad bowl, combine the baby spinach, sliced strawberries, and sliced almonds.

2. In a small bowl, whisk together the white wine vinegar, honey, Dijon mustard, olive oil, poppy seeds, salt, and pepper until well combined.

3. Drizzle the poppy seed vinaigrette over the salad and toss gently to coat.

4. Serve immediately.

Nutrition Facts: Calories 150 | Total Fat 10g | Saturated Fat 1g | Cholesterol 0mg | Sodium 260mg | Total Carbohydrates 14g | Dietary Fiber 3g | Total Sugars 9g | Protein 4g

This refreshing salad combines the sweetness of strawberries with the crunch of almonds and the tanginess of the poppy seed vinaigrette, making it a delicious and anti-inflammatory option.

3. Arugula and Fennel Salad with Citrus Vinaigrette

🕐 **Preparation: 15 minutes**

🍳 **Cook Time: 0 minutes**

✓ **Total Time: 15 minutes**

👨‍🍳 **Serves: 4**

5 oz arugula
- 1 fennel bulb, thinly sliced
- 1 orange, segmented
- 2 tablespoons olive oil
- 2 tablespoons orange juice
- 1 tablespoon white wine vinegar
- 1 teaspoon Dijon mustard
- 1 teaspoon honey
- 1/4 teaspoon salt
- 1/4 teaspoon black pepper

1. In a large salad bowl, combine the arugula, sliced fennel, and orange segments.

2. In a small bowl, whisk together the olive oil, orange juice, white wine vinegar, Dijon mustard, honey, salt, and pepper until well combined.

3. Drizzle the citrus vinaigrette over the salad and toss gently to coat.

4. Serve immediately.

Nutrition Facts: Calories 120 | Total Fat 7g | Saturated Fat 1g | Cholesterol 0mg | Sodium 260mg | Total Carbohydrates 13g | Dietary Fiber 3g | Total Sugars 8g | Protein 2g

This refreshing salad features the crunch of fennel, the bitterness of arugula, and the sweetness of orange, all dressed in a tangy citrus vinaigrette. It's a great anti-inflammatory option that's packed with nutrients.

4. Mixed Greens with Blueberries, Almonds, and Balsamic Vinaigrette

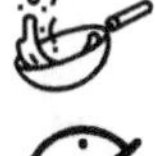 **Preparation: 10 minutes**

 **Cook Time: 0 minutes**

Total Time: 10 minutes

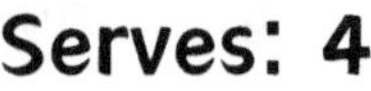 **Serves: 4**

5 oz mixed greens (such as spinach, arugula, and kale)
- 1 cup fresh blueberries
- 1/4 cup sliced almonds
- 2 tablespoons balsamic vinegar
- 1 tablespoon olive oil
- 1 teaspoon Dijon mustard
- 1 teaspoon honey
- 1/4 teaspoon salt
- 1/4 teaspoon black pepper

1. In a large salad bowl, combine the mixed greens, fresh blueberries, and sliced almonds.

2. In a small bowl, whisk together the balsamic vinegar, olive oil, Dijon mustard, honey, salt, and pepper until well combined.

3. Drizzle the balsamic vinaigrette over the salad and toss gently to coat.

4. Serve immediately.

Nutrition Facts: Calories 130 | Total Fat 8g | Saturated Fat 1g | Cholesterol 0mg | Sodium 260mg | Total Carbohydrates 12g | Dietary Fiber 3g | Total Sugars 8g | Protein 3g

This salad is a delightful blend of bitter greens, sweet blueberries, and crunchy almonds, all dressed in a tangy balsamic vinaigrette. It's a great anti-inflammatory option that's packed with antioxidants and healthy fats.

 **Preparation: 20 minutes**

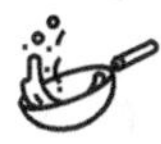 **Cook Time: 30 minutes**

 **Total Time: 50 minutes**

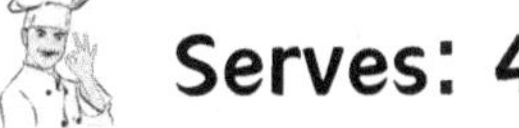 **Serves: 4**

3 medium beets, peeled and cut into 1-inch cubes
- 2 tablespoons olive oil, divided
- 1/4 teaspoon salt
- 1/4 teaspoon black pepper
- 5 oz baby kale
- 2 oz crumbled goat cheese
- 2 tablespoons balsamic vinegar
- 1 tablespoon honey
- 1 teaspoon Dijon mustard

5. Baby Kale and Roasted Beet Salad with Goat Cheese

1. Preheat the oven to 400°F. Toss the cubed beets with 1 tablespoon of olive oil, salt, and pepper. Spread the beets on a baking sheet and roast for 30 minutes, or until tender.

2. In a large salad bowl, combine the roasted beets and baby kale.

3. In a small bowl, whisk together the remaining 1 tablespoon of olive oil, balsamic vinegar, honey, and Dijon mustard.

4. Drizzle the balsamic vinaigrette over the salad and toss gently to coat.

5. Top the salad with the crumbled goat cheese and serve immediately.

Nutrition Facts: Calories 160 | Total Fat 9g | Saturated Fat 3g | Cholesterol 10mg | Sodium 320mg | Total Carbohydrates 16g | Dietary Fiber 4g | Total Sugars 10g | Protein 6g

This salad is a delicious and anti-inflammatory combination of nutrient-dense baby kale, sweet roasted beets, and creamy goat cheese, all dressed in a tangy balsamic vinaigrette.

 **Preparation: 15 minutes**

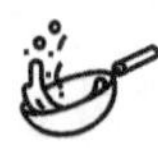 **Cook Time: 0 minutes**

 **Total Time: 15 minutes**

 **Serves: 4**

5 oz watercress, stems removed
- 2 oranges, segmented
- 1/4 cup chopped walnuts
- 2 tablespoons walnut oil
- 1 tablespoon apple cider vinegar
- 1 teaspoon Dijon mustard
- 1 teaspoon honey
- 1/4 teaspoon salt
- 1/4 teaspoon black pepper

6. Watercress and Orange Salad with Walnut Dressing

1. In a large salad bowl, combine the watercress, orange segments, and chopped walnuts.

2. In a small bowl, whisk together the walnut oil, apple cider vinegar, Dijon mustard, honey, salt, and pepper until well combined.

3. Drizzle the walnut dressing over the salad and toss gently to coat.

4. Serve immediately.

Nutrition Facts: Calories 140 | Total Fat 10g | Saturated Fat 1g | Cholesterol 0mg | Sodium 260mg | Total Carbohydrates 11g | Dietary Fiber 3g | Total Sugars 7g | Protein 3g

This refreshing salad features the peppery bite of watercress, the sweetness of oranges, and the crunch of walnuts, all dressed in a tangy walnut vinaigrette. It's a great anti-inflammatory option that's packed with vitamins and healthy fats.

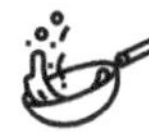 **Preparation: 15 minutes**

 **Cook Time: 0 minutes**

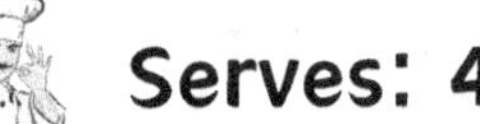 **Total Time: 15 minutes**

Serves: 4

1 bunch Swiss chard, stems removed and leaves chopped
- 1 cup pomegranate arils
- 1/4 cup crumbled feta cheese
- 2 tablespoons olive oil
- 2 tablespoons balsamic vinegar
- 1 teaspoon Dijon mustard
- 1 teaspoon honey
- 1/4 teaspoon salt
- 1/4 teaspoon black pepper

7. Swiss Chard Salad with Pomegranate and Feta

1. In a large salad bowl, combine the chopped Swiss chard, pomegranate arils, and crumbled feta cheese.

2. In a small bowl, whisk together the olive oil, balsamic vinegar, Dijon mustard, honey, salt, and pepper until well combined.

3. Drizzle the balsamic vinaigrette over the salad and toss gently to coat.

4. Serve immediately.

Nutrition Facts: Calories 160 | Total Fat 10g | Saturated Fat 3g | Cholesterol 15mg | Sodium 320mg | Total Carbohydrates 14g | Dietary Fiber 3g | Total Sugars 9g | Protein 5g

This vibrant salad features the earthy flavor of Swiss chard, the sweetness of pomegranate, and the tangy creaminess of feta, all dressed in a balsamic vinaigrette. It's a great anti-inflammatory option that's packed with vitamins and antioxidants.

8. Mustard Greens with Apple Cider Vinaigrette

 **Preparation: 10 minutes**

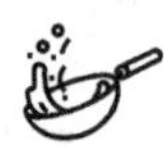 **Cook Time: 0 minutes**

 **Total Time: 10 minutes**

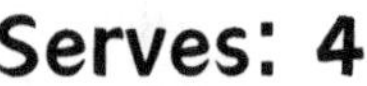 **Serves: 4**

5 oz mustard greens, stems removed and leaves chopped
- 1 apple, diced
- 2 tablespoons apple cider vinegar
- 1 tablespoon olive oil
- 1 teaspoon Dijon mustard
- 1 teaspoon honey
- 1/4 teaspoon salt
- 1/4 teaspoon black pepper

1. In a large salad bowl, combine the chopped mustard greens and diced apple.

2. In a small bowl, whisk together the apple cider vinegar, olive oil, Dijon mustard, honey, salt, and pepper until well combined.

3. Drizzle the apple cider vinaigrette over the salad and toss gently to coat.

4. Serve immediately.

Nutrition Facts: Calories 90 | Total Fat 5g | Saturated Fat 1g | Cholesterol 0mg | Sodium 260mg | Total Carbohydrates 10g | Dietary Fiber 2g | Total Sugars 6g | Protein 2g

This salad features the peppery bite of mustard greens, the sweetness of apples, and a tangy apple cider vinaigrette. It's a great anti-inflammatory option that's packed with vitamins and antioxidants.

 **Preparation: 15 minutes**

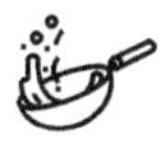 **Cook Time: 0 minutes**

 **Total Time: 15 minutes**

Serves: 4

4 cups shredded red cabbage
- 1 carrot, grated
- 2 tablespoons apple cider vinegar
- 1 tablespoon olive oil
- 1 tablespoon grated fresh ginger
- 1 teaspoon honey
- 1/4 teaspoon salt
- 1/4 teaspoon black pepper

9. Red Cabbage Slaw with Carrot and Ginger Dressing

1. In a large bowl, combine the shredded red cabbage and grated carrot.

2. In a small bowl, whisk together the apple cider vinegar, olive oil, grated ginger, honey, salt, and pepper until well combined.

3. Pour the carrot and ginger dressing over the cabbage slaw and toss to coat.

4. Serve immediately or refrigerate until ready to serve.

Nutrition Facts: Calories 80 | Total Fat 4g | Saturated Fat 1g | Cholesterol 0mg | Sodium 260mg | Total Carbohydrates 10g | Dietary Fiber 2g | Total Sugars 6g | Protein 1g

This vibrant slaw features the crunch of red cabbage and carrots, all dressed in a tangy and flavorful carrot and ginger dressing. It's a great anti-inflammatory option that's packed with vitamins and antioxidants.

10. Brussels Sprout Caesar Salad

 **Preparation: 15 minutes**

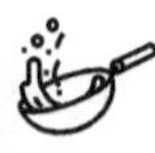 **Cook Time: 0 minutes**

 **Total Time: 15 minutes**

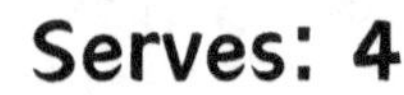 **Serves: 4**

1 lb Brussels sprouts, trimmed and shredded
- 1/4 cup grated Parmesan cheese
- 2 tablespoons olive oil
- 2 tablespoons lemon juice
- 1 tablespoon Dijon mustard
- 1 garlic clove, minced
- 1/4 teaspoon salt
- 1/4 teaspoon black pepper
- 2 tablespoons toasted breadcrumbs (optional)

1. In a large salad bowl, combine the shredded Brussels sprouts and grated Parmesan cheese.

2. In a small bowl, whisk together the olive oil, lemon juice, Dijon mustard, minced garlic, salt, and pepper until well combined.

3. Drizzle the Caesar-style dressing over the Brussels sprout salad and toss to coat.

4. Sprinkle the toasted breadcrumbs over the top, if using.

5. Serve immediately.

Nutrition Facts: Calories 130 | Total Fat 9g | Saturated Fat 2g | Cholesterol 5mg | Sodium 320mg | Total Carbohydrates 9g | Dietary Fiber 3g | Total Sugars 2g | Protein 6g

This Brussels sprout-based Caesar salad is a delicious and anti-inflammatory twist on a classic. The shredded Brussels sprouts provide a crunchy base, while the Parmesan and Caesar-style dressing add a creamy, tangy flavor.

🕐 **Preparation: 20 minutes**

Cook Time: 0 minutes

Total Time: 20 minutes

Serves: 4

1 bunch collard greens, stems removed and leaves chopped
- 1 red bell pepper, thinly sliced
- 1/4 cup roasted peanuts
- 2 tablespoons creamy peanut butter
- 2 tablespoons rice vinegar
- 1 tablespoon soy sauce
- 1 teaspoon honey
- 1 teaspoon sesame oil
- 1/4 teaspoon red pepper flakes (or more to taste)
- 1/4 teaspoon salt

11. Collard Greens Salad with Spicy Peanut Dressing

1. In a large salad bowl, combine the chopped collard greens, sliced red bell pepper, and roasted peanuts.

2. In a small bowl, whisk together the peanut butter, rice vinegar, soy sauce, honey, sesame oil, red pepper flakes, and salt until well combined.

3. Drizzle the spicy peanut dressing over the collard greens salad and toss to coat.

4. Serve immediately.

Nutrition Facts: Calories 160 | Total Fat 10g | Saturated Fat 1.5g | Cholesterol 0mg | Sodium 360mg | Total Carbohydrates 13g | Dietary Fiber 4g | Total Sugars 5g | Protein 7g

This nutrient-dense salad features the bitterness of collard greens, the crunch of bell peppers and peanuts, and a spicy peanut dressing that adds a delicious flavor. It's a great anti-inflammatory option that's packed with vitamins and healthy fats.

 **Preparation: 15 minutes**

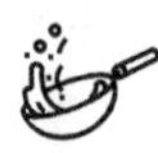 **Cook Time: 0 minutes**

 **Total Time: 15 minutes**

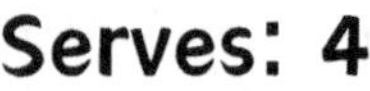 **Serves: 4**

1 head radicchio, leaves torn into bite-sized pieces
- 2 heads endive, leaves separated
- 2 tablespoons olive oil
- 2 tablespoons lemon juice
- 1 tablespoon honey
- 1 teaspoon Dijon mustard
- 1/4 teaspoon salt
- 1/4 teaspoon black pepper

12. Radicchio and Endive Salad with Lemon-Honey Dressing

1. In a large salad bowl, combine the torn radicchio leaves and endive leaves.

2. In a small bowl, whisk together the olive oil, lemon juice, honey, Dijon mustard, salt, and pepper until well combined.

3. Drizzle the lemon-honey dressing over the radicchio and endive salad and toss gently to coat.

4. Serve immediately.

Nutrition Facts: Calories 100 | Total Fat 6g | Saturated Fat 1g | Cholesterol 0mg | Sodium 260mg | Total Carbohydrates 11g | Dietary Fiber 3g | Total Sugars 6g | Protein 2g

This salad features the bitterness of radicchio and endive, balanced by the sweetness of the lemon-honey dressing. It's a great anti-inflammatory option that's packed with vitamins and antioxidants.

 **Preparation: 10 minutes**

 **Cook Time: 0 minutes**

Total Time: 10 minutes

Serves: 4

6 cups chopped romaine lettuce
- 1 avocado, diced
- 1/4 cup roasted pumpkin seeds
- 2 tablespoons olive oil
- 2 tablespoons lime juice
- 1 tablespoon honey
- 1 teaspoon Dijon mustard
- 1/4 teaspoon salt
- 1/4 teaspoon black pepper

13. Romaine with Avocado, Pumpkin Seeds, and Lime Dressing

1. In a large salad bowl, combine the chopped romaine lettuce, diced avocado, and roasted pumpkin seeds.

2. In a small bowl, whisk together the olive oil, lime juice, honey, Dijon mustard, salt, and pepper until well combined.

3. Drizzle the lime dressing over the salad and toss gently to coat.

4. Serve immediately.

Nutrition Facts: Calories 180 | Total Fat 14g | Saturated Fat 2g | Cholesterol 0mg | Sodium 260mg | Total Carbohydrates 12g | Dietary Fiber 5g | Total Sugars 5g | Protein 4g

This refreshing salad features the crunch of romaine lettuce, the creaminess of avocado, and the nutty flavor of roasted pumpkin seeds, all dressed in a tangy lime vinaigrette. It's a great anti-inflammatory option that's packed with healthy fats and nutrients.

14. Butter Lettuce with Pear, Walnut, and Gorgonzola

 **Preparation: 10 minutes**

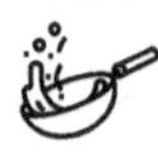 **Cook Time: 0 minutes**

 **Total Time: 10 minutes**

 **Serves: 4**

6 cups butter lettuce, torn into bite-sized pieces
- 1 pear, thinly sliced
- 1/4 cup crumbled Gorgonzola cheese
- 1/4 cup chopped walnuts
- 2 tablespoons olive oil
- 2 tablespoons balsamic vinegar
- 1 teaspoon honey
- 1/4 teaspoon salt
- 1/4 teaspoon black pepper

1. In a large salad bowl, combine the torn butter lettuce, sliced pear, crumbled Gorgonzola cheese, and chopped walnuts.

2. In a small bowl, whisk together the olive oil, balsamic vinegar, honey, salt, and pepper until well combined.

3. Drizzle the balsamic vinaigrette over the salad and toss gently to coat.

4. Serve immediately.

Nutrition Facts: Calories 180 | Total Fat 14g | Saturated Fat 3g | Cholesterol 10mg | Sodium 320mg | Total Carbohydrates 12g | Dietary Fiber 3g | Total Sugars 7g | Protein 5g

This salad features the delicate texture of butter lettuce, the sweetness of pear, the creaminess of Gorgonzola, and the crunch of walnuts, all dressed in a tangy balsamic vinaigrette. It's a great anti-inflammatory option that's packed with healthy fats and nutrients.

15. Bok Choy Salad with Sesame Ginger Dressing

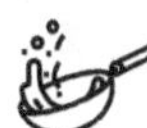 **Preparation: 15 minutes**

 **Cook Time: 0 minutes**

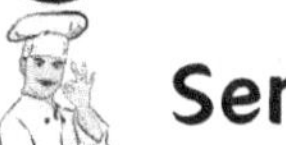 **Total Time: 15 minutes**

Serves: 4

1 lb bok choy, thinly sliced
- 1 red bell pepper, thinly sliced
- 1/4 cup toasted sesame seeds
- 2 tablespoons rice vinegar
- 2 tablespoons sesame oil
- 1 tablespoon soy sauce
- 1 tablespoon grated fresh ginger
- 1 teaspoon honey
- 1/4 teaspoon salt
- 1/4 teaspoon black pepper

1. In a large salad bowl, combine the thinly sliced bok choy, sliced red bell pepper, and toasted sesame seeds.

2. In a small bowl, whisk together the rice vinegar, sesame oil, soy sauce, grated ginger, honey, salt, and pepper until well combined.

3. Drizzle the sesame ginger dressing over the bok choy salad and toss gently to coat.

4. Serve immediately.

Nutrition Facts: Calories 120 | Total Fat 8g | Saturated Fat 1g | Cholesterol 0mg | Sodium 360mg | Total Carbohydrates 10g | Dietary Fiber 3g | Total Sugars 4g | Protein 4g

This refreshing salad features the crunch of bok choy and bell peppers, the nutty flavor of toasted sesame seeds, and a tangy sesame ginger dressing. It's a great anti-inflammatory option that's packed with vitamins and antioxidants.

 **Preparation: 10 minutes**

 **Cook Time: 5 minutes**

 **Total Time: 15 minutes**

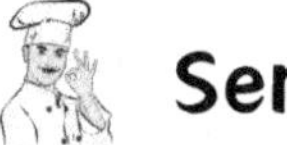 **Serves: 4**

 6 cups dandelion greens, washed and torn into bite-sized pieces
- 3 slices bacon, cooked and crumbled
- 2 tablespoons bacon fat (reserved from cooking the bacon)
- 2 tablespoons apple cider vinegar
- 1 teaspoon Dijon mustard
- 1 teaspoon honey
- 1/4 teaspoon salt
- 1/4 teaspoon black pepper

16. Dandelion Greens with Warm Bacon Vinaigrette

1. In a large salad bowl, combine the torn dandelion greens and crumbled bacon.

2. In a small saucepan, heat the reserved bacon fat over medium heat. Whisk in the apple cider vinegar, Dijon mustard, honey, salt, and pepper until well combined.

3. Immediately pour the warm bacon vinaigrette over the dandelion greens and toss to coat.

4. Serve the salad while the dressing is still warm.

Nutrition Facts: Calories 110 | Total Fat 8g | Saturated Fat 2g | Cholesterol 10mg | Sodium 320mg | Total Carbohydrates 6g | Dietary Fiber 2g | Total Sugars 3g | Protein 4g

This salad features the bitterness of dandelion greens, balanced by the richness of the warm bacon vinaigrette. It's a great anti-inflammatory option that's packed with vitamins and antioxidants.

 **Preparation: 15 minutes**

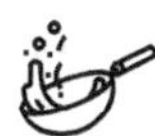 **Cook Time: 15 minutes**

 **Total Time: 30 minutes**

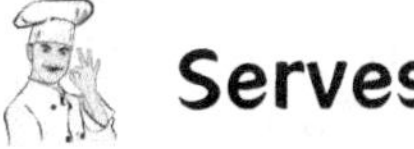 **Serves: 4**

5 oz mesclun mix (a blend of baby greens)
- 1 cup cooked quinoa
- 2 tablespoons tahini
- 2 tablespoons lemon juice
- 1 tablespoon olive oil
- 1 tablespoon water
- 1 garlic clove, minced
- 1 teaspoon honey
- 1/4 teaspoon salt
- 1/4 teaspoon black pepper

17. Mesclun Mix with Quinoa and Tahini Dressing

1. In a large salad bowl, combine the mesclun mix and cooked quinoa.

2. In a small bowl, whisk together the tahini, lemon juice, olive oil, water, minced garlic, honey, salt, and pepper until well combined.

3. Drizzle the tahini dressing over the salad and toss gently to coat.

4. Serve immediately.

Nutrition Facts: Calories 180 | Total Fat 9g | Saturated Fat 1g | Cholesterol 0mg | Sodium 260mg | Total Carbohydrates 19g | Dietary Fiber 3g | Total Sugars 4g | Protein 6g

This salad features a nutrient-dense blend of mesclun greens and protein-rich quinoa, all dressed in a creamy tahini dressing. It's a great anti-inflammatory option that's packed with fiber, vitamins, and healthy fats.

18. Baby Spinach with Cranberries, Pecans, and Maple Vinaigrette

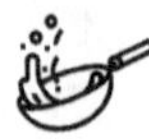 **Preparation: 10 minutes**

 **Cook Time: 0 minutes**

 **Total Time: 10 minutes**

Serves: 4

5 oz baby spinach
- 1/2 cup dried cranberries
- 1/4 cup chopped pecans
- 2 tablespoons olive oil
- 2 tablespoons maple syrup
- 1 tablespoon apple cider vinegar
- 1 teaspoon Dijon mustard
- 1/4 teaspoon salt
- 1/4 teaspoon black pepper

1. In a large salad bowl, combine the baby spinach, dried cranberries, and chopped pecans.

2. In a small bowl, whisk together the olive oil, maple syrup, apple cider vinegar, Dijon mustard, salt, and pepper until well combined.

3. Drizzle the maple vinaigrette over the salad and toss gently to coat.

4. Serve immediately.

Nutrition Facts: Calories 170 | Total Fat 11g | Saturated Fat 1g | Cholesterol 0mg | Sodium 260mg | Total Carbohydrates 16g | Dietary Fiber 3g | Total Sugars 11g | Protein 3g

This salad features the sweetness of dried cranberries and maple syrup, the crunch of pecans, and the bitterness of baby spinach, all dressed in a tangy maple vinaigrette. It's a great anti-inflammatory option that's packed with vitamins and healthy fats.

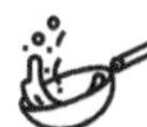 **Preparation: 15 minutes**

 **Cook Time: 0 minutes**

Total Time: 15 minutes

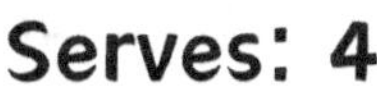 **Serves: 4**

 1 bunch kale, stems removed and leaves chopped
- 2 cups broccoli florets, chopped
- 2 tablespoons olive oil
- 2 tablespoons lemon juice
- 1 garlic clove, minced
- 1 teaspoon Dijon mustard
- 1 teaspoon honey
- 1/4 teaspoon salt
- 1/4 teaspoon black pepper

19. Kale and Broccoli Salad with Lemon-Garlic Dressing

1. In a large salad bowl, combine the chopped kale and broccoli florets.

2. In a small bowl, whisk together the olive oil, lemon juice, minced garlic, Dijon mustard, honey, salt, and pepper until well combined.

3. Drizzle the lemon-garlic dressing over the kale and broccoli salad and toss to coat.

4. Serve immediately.

Nutrition Facts: Calories 120 | Total Fat 7g | Saturated Fat 1g | Cholesterol 0mg | Sodium 260mg | Total Carbohydrates 12g | Dietary Fiber 3g | Total Sugars 4g | Protein 4g

This salad features the nutrient-dense combination of kale and broccoli, dressed in a tangy lemon-garlic vinaigrette. It's a great anti-inflammatory option that's packed with vitamins, minerals, and antioxidants.

20. Napa Cabbage with Miso-Ginger Dressing

 **Preparation: 10 minutes**

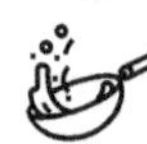 **Cook Time: 0 minutes**

 **Total Time: 10 minutes**

Serves: 4

1 head napa cabbage, thinly sliced
- 2 tablespoons white miso paste
- 2 tablespoons rice vinegar
- 1 tablespoon sesame oil
- 1 tablespoon grated fresh ginger
- 1 teaspoon honey
- 1/4 teaspoon salt
- 1/4 teaspoon black pepper

1. In a large salad bowl, toss the thinly sliced napa cabbage.

2. In a small bowl, whisk together the white miso paste, rice vinegar, sesame oil, grated ginger, honey, salt, and pepper until well combined.

3. Drizzle the miso-ginger dressing over the napa cabbage and toss to coat.

4. Serve immediately.

Nutrition Facts: Calories 90 | Total Fat 5g | Saturated Fat 1g | Cholesterol 0mg | Sodium 360mg | Total Carbohydrates 10g | Dietary Fiber 3g | Total Sugars 4g | Protein 3g

This salad features the crunchy texture of napa cabbage, dressed in a flavorful miso-ginger vinaigrette. It's a great anti-inflammatory option that's packed with vitamins, minerals, and probiotics from the miso.

Preparation: 15 minutes

Cook Time: 10 minutes

Total Time: 25 minutes

Serves: 4

1 lb boneless, skinless chicken breasts
- 1 avocado, diced
- 5 oz mixed greens
- 1/4 cup diced red onion
- 2 tablespoons olive oil
- 2 tablespoons lime juice
- 1 teaspoon Dijon mustard
- 1 teaspoon honey
- 1/4 teaspoon salt
- 1/4 teaspoon black pepper

1. Grilled Chicken and Avocado Salad with Lime Vinaigrette

1. Preheat grill or grill pan to medium-high heat. Season the chicken breasts with salt and pepper.

2. Grill the chicken for 5-7 minutes per side, or until cooked through. Allow to cool slightly, then slice or shred the chicken.

3. In a large salad bowl, combine the grilled chicken, diced avocado, mixed greens, and diced red onion.

4. In a small bowl, whisk together the olive oil, lime juice, Dijon mustard, honey, salt, and pepper.

5. Drizzle the lime vinaigrette over the salad and toss gently to coat.

6. Serve immediately.

Nutrition Facts: Calories 320 | Total Fat 16g | Saturated Fat 2.5g | Cholesterol 75mg | Sodium 360mg | Total Carbohydrates 12g | Dietary Fiber 5g | Total Sugars 6g | Protein 32g

This salad is a delicious and filling option, featuring grilled chicken, creamy avocado, and a tangy lime vinaigrette. It's a great anti-inflammatory choice that's packed with protein, healthy fats, and vitamins.

 **Preparation: 20 minutes**

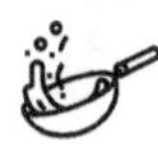 **Cook Time: 15 minutes**

 **Total Time: 35 minutes**

 **Serves: 4**

 1 cup cooked quinoa
- 1 (15 oz) can black beans, rinsed and drained
- 1 cup diced cucumber
- 1/2 cup diced red bell pepper
- 1/4 cup diced red onion
- 2 tablespoons olive oil
- 2 tablespoons lime juice
- 1 teaspoon ground cumin
- 1 teaspoon honey
- 1/4 teaspoon salt
- 1/4 teaspoon black pepper

2. Quinoa and Black Bean Salad with Cumin-Lime Dressing

1. In a large bowl, combine the cooked quinoa, black beans, diced cucumber, red bell pepper, and red onion.

2. In a small bowl, whisk together the olive oil, lime juice, ground cumin, honey, salt, and pepper.

3. Drizzle the cumin-lime dressing over the quinoa and black bean salad, and toss gently to coat.

4. Serve immediately or refrigerate until ready to serve.

Nutrition Facts: Calories 250 | Total Fat 8g | Saturated Fat 1g | Cholesterol 0mg | Sodium 360mg | Total Carbohydrates 35g | Dietary Fiber 8g | Total Sugars 5g | Protein 9g

This salad is a nutritious and flavorful combination of protein-rich quinoa and black beans, along with fresh vegetables, all dressed in a tangy cumin-lime vinaigrette. It's a great anti-inflammatory option that's packed with fiber, vitamins, and minerals.

3. Salmon and Asparagus Salad with Dijon Vinaigrette

 **Preparation: 15 minutes**

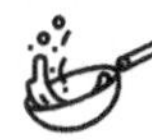 **Cook Time: 10 minutes**

 **Total Time: 25 minutes**

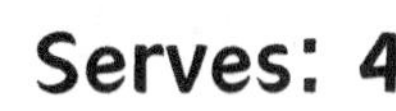 **Serves: 4**

 1 lb salmon fillets
- 1 lb asparagus, trimmed and cut into 1-inch pieces
- 5 oz mixed greens
- 2 tablespoons olive oil
- 2 tablespoons white wine vinegar
- 1 tablespoon Dijon mustard
- 1 teaspoon honey
- 1/4 teaspoon salt
- 1/4 teaspoon black pepper

1. Preheat oven to 400°F. Place the salmon fillets on a baking sheet and roast for 10-12 minutes, or until cooked through. Allow to cool slightly, then flake the salmon into large chunks.

2. In a large pot of boiling water, blanch the asparagus for 2-3 minutes until tender-crisp. Drain and rinse with cold water.

3. In a large salad bowl, combine the flaked salmon, blanched asparagus, and mixed greens.

4. In a small bowl, whisk together the olive oil, white wine vinegar, Dijon mustard, honey, salt, and pepper.

5. Drizzle the Dijon vinaigrette over the salad and toss gently to coat.

6. Serve immediately.

Nutrition Facts: Calories 280 | Total Fat 15g | Saturated Fat 2.5g | Cholesterol 60mg | Sodium 420mg | Total Carbohydrates 8g | Dietary Fiber 3g | Total Sugars 4g | Protein 28g

This salad features the omega-3 rich salmon, paired with tender-crisp asparagus and a tangy Dijon vinaigrette. It's a delicious and anti-inflammatory option that's packed with protein, healthy fats, and vitamins.

 **Preparation: 15 minutes**

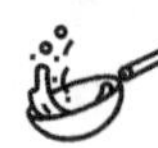 **Cook Time: 0 minutes**

 **Total Time: 15 minutes**

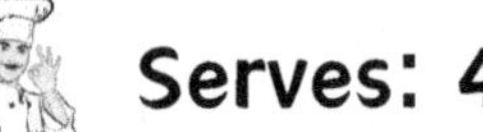 **Serves: 4**

5 oz baby spinach
- 1 cup cooked turkey breast, diced
- 1/2 cup dried cranberries
- 1/4 cup toasted pecans
- 2 tablespoons olive oil
- 2 tablespoons cranberry juice
- 1 tablespoon balsamic vinegar
- 1 teaspoon Dijon mustard
- 1 teaspoon honey
- 1/4 teaspoon salt
- 1/4 teaspoon black pepper

4. Turkey and Spinach Salad with Cranberry Dressing

1. In a large salad bowl, combine the baby spinach, diced turkey, dried cranberries, and toasted pecans.

2. In a small bowl, whisk together the olive oil, cranberry juice, balsamic vinegar, Dijon mustard, honey, salt, and pepper.

3. Drizzle the cranberry dressing over the salad and toss gently to coat.

4. Serve immediately.

Nutrition Facts: Calories 240 | Total Fat 12g | Saturated Fat 2g | Cholesterol 45mg | Sodium 360mg | Total Carbohydrates 18g | Dietary Fiber 3g | Total Sugars 13g | Protein 18g

This salad features the lean protein of turkey, the crunch of pecans, and the sweetness of dried cranberries, all dressed in a tangy cranberry vinaigrette. It's a great anti-inflammatory option that's packed with vitamins and antioxidants.

5. Tofu and Edamame Salad with Sesame Dressing

 **Preparation: 15 minutes**

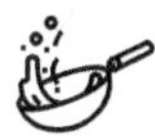 **Cook Time: 0 minutes**

 **Total Time: 15 minutes**

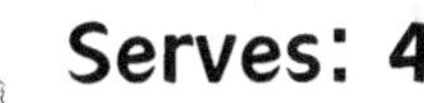 **Serves: 4**

1 block firm tofu, cubed
- 1 cup shelled edamame
- 2 cups mixed greens
- 2 tablespoons sesame oil
- 2 tablespoons rice vinegar
- 1 tablespoon soy sauce
- 1 teaspoon sesame seeds
- 1 teaspoon honey
- 1/4 teaspoon salt
- 1/4 teaspoon black pepper

1. In a large salad bowl, combine the cubed tofu, shelled edamame, and mixed greens.

2. In a small bowl, whisk together the sesame oil, rice vinegar, soy sauce, sesame seeds, honey, salt, and pepper.

3. Drizzle the sesame dressing over the salad and toss gently to coat.

4. Serve immediately.

Nutrition Facts: Calories 200 | Total Fat 12g | Saturated Fat 2g | Cholesterol 0mg | Sodium 420mg | Total Carbohydrates 12g | Dietary Fiber 4g | Total Sugars 4g | Protein 14g

This salad features the plant-based protein of tofu and edamame, along with a flavorful sesame dressing. It's a great anti-inflammatory option that's packed with fiber, vitamins, and healthy fats.

6. Shrimp and Mango Salad with Cilantro-Lime Dressing

 **Preparation: 20 minutes**

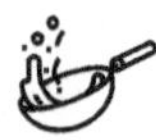 **Cook Time: 5 minutes**

 **Total Time: 25 minutes**

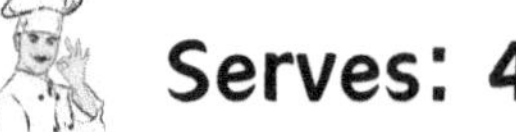 **Serves: 4**

- 1 lb cooked shrimp, peeled and deveined
- 1 mango, diced
- 1 avocado, diced
- 5 oz mixed greens
- 2 tablespoons olive oil
- 2 tablespoons lime juice
- 2 tablespoons chopped fresh cilantro
- 1 teaspoon honey
- 1/4 teaspoon salt
- 1/4 teaspoon black pepper

1. In a large salad bowl, combine the cooked shrimp, diced mango, diced avocado, and mixed greens.

2. In a small bowl, whisk together the olive oil, lime juice, chopped cilantro, honey, salt, and pepper.

3. Drizzle the cilantro-lime dressing over the salad and toss gently to coat.

4. Serve immediately.

Nutrition Facts: Calories 280 | Total Fat 14g | Saturated Fat 2g | Cholesterol 170mg | Sodium 420mg | Total Carbohydrates 18g | Dietary Fiber 5g | Total Sugars 12g | Protein 22g

This salad features the sweetness of mango, the creaminess of avocado, and the protein-rich shrimp, all dressed in a tangy cilantro-lime vinaigrette. It's a delicious and anti-inflammatory option that's packed with vitamins, minerals, and healthy fats.

7. Hard-Boiled Egg and Kale Salad with Lemon-Dill Dressing

 **Preparation: 15 minutes**

 **Cook Time: 10 minutes**

Total Time: 25 minutes

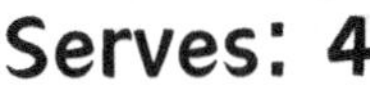 **Serves: 4**

4 hard-boiled eggs, peeled and sliced
- 1 bunch kale, stems removed and leaves chopped
- 1/2 cup cherry tomatoes, halved
- 2 tablespoons olive oil
- 2 tablespoons lemon juice
- 1 tablespoon chopped fresh dill
- 1 teaspoon Dijon mustard
- 1 teaspoon honey
- 1/4 teaspoon salt
- 1/4 teaspoon black pepper

1. In a large salad bowl, combine the sliced hard-boiled eggs, chopped kale, and halved cherry tomatoes.

2. In a small bowl, whisk together the olive oil, lemon juice, chopped dill, Dijon mustard, honey, salt, and pepper.

3. Drizzle the lemon-dill dressing over the salad and toss gently to coat.

4. Serve immediately.

Nutrition Facts: Calories 190 | Total Fat 12g | Saturated Fat 2.5g | Cholesterol 185mg | Sodium 360mg | Total Carbohydrates 10g | Dietary Fiber 3g | Total Sugars 4g | Protein 12g

This salad features the protein-rich hard-boiled eggs, the nutrient-dense kale, and the freshness of cherry tomatoes, all dressed in a tangy lemon-dill vinaigrette. It's a great anti-inflammatory option that's packed with vitamins, minerals, and healthy fats.

Preparation: 10 minutes

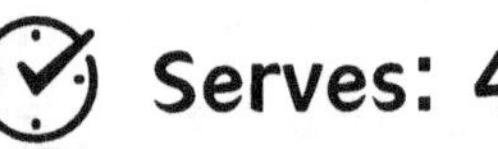

Total Time: 10 minutes

Serves: 4

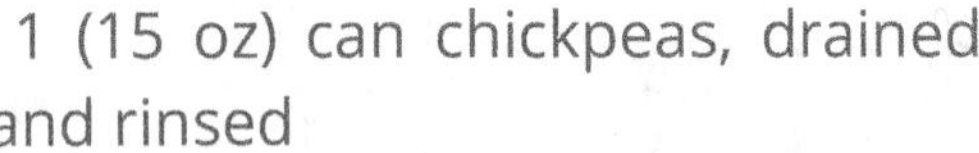

1 (15 oz) can chickpeas, drained and rinsed
- 1 (5 oz) can tuna, drained
- 1/4 cup diced red onion
- 1/4 cup diced celery
- 2 tbsp chopped parsley
- 2 tbsp lemon juice
- 2 tbsp tahini
- 1 tbsp olive oil
- 1 tsp Dijon mustard
- 1 garlic clove, minced
- Salt and pepper to taste

8. Tuna and Chickpea Salad with Lemon-Tahini Dressing

1. In a medium bowl, combine the chickpeas, tuna, red onion, celery, and parsley. Gently mix to combine.

2. In a small bowl, whisk together the lemon juice, tahini, olive oil, Dijon mustard, and garlic. Season with salt and pepper.

3. Pour the lemon-tahini dressing over the chickpea and tuna salad and toss gently to coat.

4. Serve the salad chilled or at room temperature. It can be served on a bed of greens, stuffed into tomatoes or avocados, or scooped onto crackers or bread.

Nutrition Facts: Calories 190, Total Fat 9g, Saturated Fat 1g, Cholesterol 15mg, Sodium 360mg, Total Carbohydrates 16g, Dietary Fiber 5g, Total Sugars 2g, Protein 13g

 **Preparation: 15 minutes**

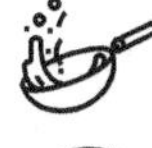 **Cook Time: 10 minutes**

 **Total Time: 25 minutes**

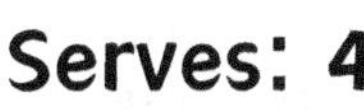 **Serves: 4**

1 lb flank steak
- 5 oz baby arugula
- 1 cup cherry tomatoes, halved
- 1/2 red onion, thinly sliced
- 1/4 cup crumbled feta cheese

Chimichurri Dressing:
- 1 cup packed fresh parsley
- 3 garlic cloves
- 2 tbsp red wine vinegar
- 1 tbsp olive oil
- 1 tsp dried oregano
- 1/4 tsp red pepper flakes
- Salt and pepper to taste

9. Grilled Steak Salad with Arugula and Chimichurri

1. Make the chimichurri dressing: In a food processor, combine the parsley, garlic, red wine vinegar, olive oil, oregano, and red pepper flakes. Pulse until well combined but still slightly chunky. Season with salt and pepper to taste.

2. Preheat grill or grill pan to medium-high heat. Season the steak with salt and pepper.

3. Grill the steak for 4-5 minutes per side, or until it reaches your desired doneness. Let the steak rest for 5 minutes, then slice it against the grain.

4. In a large salad bowl, combine the arugula, cherry tomatoes, and red onion.

5. Top the salad with the grilled steak slices and crumbled feta cheese.

6. Drizzle the chimichurri dressing over the salad and toss gently to coat.

7. Serve immediately.

Nutrition Facts: Calories 320, Total Fat 18g, Saturated Fat 5g, Cholesterol 60mg, Sodium 450mg, Total Carbohydrates 10g, Dietary Fiber 3g, Total Sugars 4g, Protein 30g

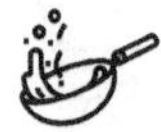 **Preparation: 15 minutes**

 **Cook Time: 20 minutes**

 **Total Time: 35 minutes**

Serves: 4

8 oz tempeh, cut into 1-inch cubes
- 2 tbsp olive oil
- 1 tsp soy sauce
- 1 tsp maple syrup
- 1/4 tsp garlic powder
- 1/4 tsp ground ginger
- 5 oz mixed greens
- 1 cup shredded red cabbage
- 1 cup shredded carrots
- 1/2 cup chopped cucumber
- 2 tbsp chopped cilantro

Peanut Sauce:
- 1/4 cup creamy peanut butter
- 2 tbsp soy sauce
- 2 tbsp rice vinegar
- 1 tbsp maple syrup
- 1 tbsp water
- 1 tsp sesame oil
- 1 garlic clove, minced
- 1/4 tsp red pepper flakes (optional)

10. Baked Tempeh Salad with Peanut Sauce

1. Preheat the oven to 400°F. Line a baking sheet with parchment paper.

2. In a bowl, toss the tempeh cubes with the olive oil, soy sauce, maple syrup, garlic powder, and ground ginger. Spread the tempeh on the prepared baking sheet and bake for 18-20 minutes, flipping halfway, until crispy.

3. In a large salad bowl, combine the mixed greens, red cabbage, carrots, cucumber, and cilantro.

4. Make the peanut sauce: In a small bowl, whisk together the peanut butter, soy sauce, rice vinegar, maple syrup, water, sesame oil, garlic, and red pepper flakes (if using).

5. Add the baked tempeh to the salad and drizzle the peanut sauce over the top. Toss gently to coat.

6. Serve the salad immediately.

Nutrition Facts: Calories 320, Total Fat 18g, Saturated Fat 3g, Cholesterol 0mg, Sodium 650mg, Total Carbohydrates 24g, Dietary Fiber 6g, Total Sugars 10g, Protein 18g

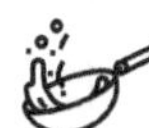 **Preparation: 15 minutes**

 **Cook Time: 10 minutes**

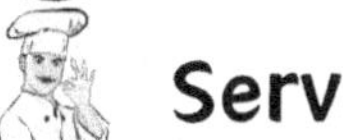 **Total Time: 25 minutes**

Serves: 4

1 lb boneless, skinless chicken breasts
- 1 tbsp olive oil
- 1 tsp dried oregano
- Salt and pepper to taste
- 6 cups chopped romaine lettuce
- 1 cup cherry tomatoes, halved
- 1/2 cup sliced cucumber
- 1/4 cup sliced red onion
- 1/4 cup pitted kalamata olives, halved
- 1/2 cup crumbled feta cheese
- 2 tbsp chopped fresh parsley

Dressing:
- 2 tbsp red wine vinegar
- 1 tbsp olive oil
- 1 tbsp lemon juice
- 1 tsp Dijon mustard
- 1 garlic clove, minced
- 1/2 tsp dried oregano
- Salt and pepper to taste

11. Greek Salad with Feta and Chicken

1. Preheat a grill or grill pan to medium-high heat.

2. Season the chicken breasts with the olive oil, dried oregano, salt, and pepper.

3. Grill the chicken for 5-6 minutes per side, or until cooked through. Let the chicken rest for 5 minutes, then slice or chop it.

4. In a large salad bowl, combine the romaine lettuce, cherry tomatoes, cucumber, red onion, kalamata olives, feta cheese, and parsley.

5. In a small bowl, whisk together the ingredients for the dressing.

6. Add the grilled chicken to the salad and drizzle the dressing over the top. Toss gently to coat.

7. Serve the Greek salad immediately.

Nutrition Facts: Calories 320, Total Fat 16g, Saturated Fat 5g, Cholesterol 90mg, Sodium 650mg, Total Carbohydrates 12g, Dietary Fiber 3g, Total Sugars 5g, Protein 32g

12. Lentil and Beet Salad with Balsamic Vinaigrette

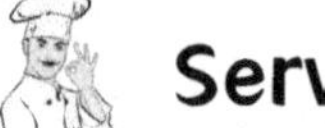

Preparation: 20 minutes

Cook Time: 20 minutes

Total Time: 40 minutes

Serves: 4

 1 cup cooked lentils
- 2 medium beets, roasted and diced
- 1 cup baby spinach
- 1/2 cup diced cucumber
- 1/4 cup crumbled feta cheese
- 2 tbsp chopped walnuts

Balsamic Vinaigrette:
- 2 tbsp balsamic vinegar
- 1 tbsp olive oil
- 1 tsp Dijon mustard
- 1 tsp honey
- 1 garlic clove, minced
- Salt and pepper to taste

1. Preheat the oven to 400°F. Wrap the beets in foil and roast for 20-25 minutes, or until tender when pierced with a fork. Let cool, then peel and dice the beets.

2. In a large salad bowl, combine the cooked lentils, roasted beets, baby spinach, diced cucumber, crumbled feta, and chopped walnuts.

3. In a small bowl, whisk together the balsamic vinegar, olive oil, Dijon mustard, honey, and minced garlic. Season with salt and pepper to taste.

4. Drizzle the balsamic vinaigrette over the salad and toss gently to coat.

5. Serve the lentil and beet salad immediately.

Nutrition Facts: Calories 220, Total Fat 12g, Saturated Fat 3g, Cholesterol 10mg, Sodium 320mg, Total Carbohydrates 20g, Dietary Fiber 7g, Total Sugars 8g, Protein 9g

 **Preparation: 15 minutes**

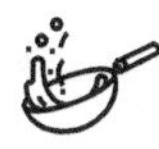 **Cook Time: 10 minutes**

 **Total Time: 25 minutes**

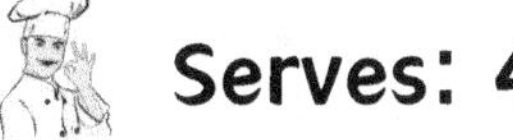 **Serves: 4**

12 oz sea scallops, patted dry
- 1 tbsp olive oil
- 5 oz mixed greens
- 1 grapefruit, segmented
- 1 orange, segmented
- 1/2 avocado, diced
- 2 tbsp toasted sliced almonds

Citrus Vinaigrette:
- 2 tbsp orange juice
- 1 tbsp grapefruit juice
- 1 tbsp white wine vinegar
- 1 tbsp olive oil
- 1 tsp Dijon mustard
- 1 tsp honey
- Salt and pepper to taste

13. Seared Scallop Salad with Citrus Vinaigrette

1. In a large skillet, heat the olive oil over medium-high heat. Season the scallops with salt and pepper.

2. Sear the scallops for 2-3 minutes per side, until golden brown and cooked through. Transfer the scallops to a plate and set aside.

3. In a small bowl, whisk together the ingredients for the citrus vinaigrette. Season with salt and pepper to taste.

4. In a large salad bowl, combine the mixed greens, grapefruit segments, orange segments, avocado, and toasted almonds.

5. Top the salad with the seared scallops and drizzle the citrus vinaigrette over the top.

6. Serve the salad immediately.

Nutrition Facts: Calories 260, Total Fat 14g, Saturated Fat 2g, Cholesterol 35mg, Sodium 380mg, Total Carbohydrates 16g, Dietary Fiber 5g, Total Sugars 9g, Protein 18g

 **Preparation: 15 minutes**

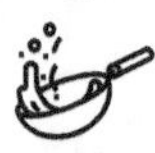 **Total Time: 15 minutes**

 **Serves: 4**

 6 cups chopped kale
- 1 apple, diced
- 1/2 cup shredded carrots
- 1/4 cup hemp seeds
- 2 tbsp dried cranberries
- 2 tbsp chopped walnuts

Apple Cider Vinaigrette:
- 2 tbsp apple cider vinegar
- 1 tbsp olive oil
- 1 tsp Dijon mustard
- 1 tsp maple syrup
- 1 garlic clove, minced
- Salt and pepper to taste

14. Hemp Seed and Kale Salad with Apple Cider Vinaigrette

1. In a large salad bowl, combine the chopped kale, diced apple, shredded carrots, hemp seeds, dried cranberries, and chopped walnuts.

2. In a small bowl, whisk together the ingredients for the apple cider vinaigrette. Season with salt and pepper to taste.

3. Drizzle the vinaigrette over the salad and toss gently to coat.

4. Serve the hemp seed and kale salad immediately.

Nutrition Facts: Calories 180, Total Fat 11g, Saturated Fat 1g, Cholesterol 0mg, Sodium 120mg, Total Carbohydrates 18g, Dietary Fiber 4g, Total Sugars 9g, Protein 6g

 **Preparation: 20 minutes**

 **Marinate Time: 30 minutes**

 **Total Time: 50 minutes**

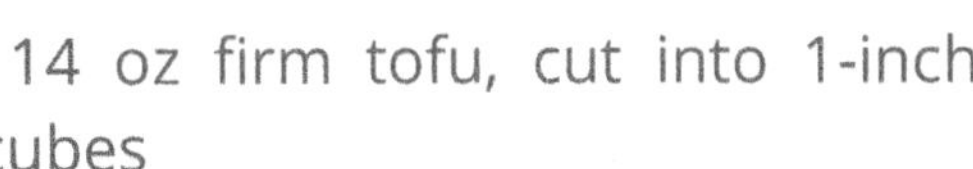 **Serves: 4**

14 oz firm tofu, cut into 1-inch cubes
- 2 tbsp white miso paste
- 2 tbsp rice vinegar
- 1 tbsp sesame oil
- 1 tbsp honey
- 1 tsp grated ginger
- 4 cups chopped bok choy
- 1 cup shredded red cabbage
- 1/2 cup shredded carrots
- 2 tbsp toasted sesame seeds
- 2 tbsp chopped green onions

Dressing:
- 2 tbsp rice vinegar
- 1 tbsp sesame oil
- 1 tbsp soy sauce
- 1 tsp honey
- 1 garlic clove, minced

15. Miso-Marinated Tofu Salad with Bok Choy

1. In a shallow dish, whisk together the miso paste, rice vinegar, sesame oil, honey, and grated ginger. Add the tofu cubes and gently toss to coat. Cover and marinate for 30 minutes, turning the tofu occasionally.

2. In a large salad bowl, combine the chopped bok choy, shredded red cabbage, and shredded carrots.

3. In a small bowl, whisk together the ingredients for the dressing.

4. Heat a large skillet or wok over medium-high heat. Add the marinated tofu and cook for 2-3 minutes per side, until lightly browned.

5. Add the cooked tofu to the salad bowl. Drizzle the dressing over the salad and toss gently to coat.

6. Sprinkle the toasted sesame seeds and chopped green onions over the top.

7. Serve the miso-marinated tofu salad immediately.

Nutrition Facts: Calories 220, Total Fat 12g, Saturated Fat 2g, Cholesterol 0mg, Sodium 580mg, Total Carbohydrates 18g, Dietary Fiber 4g, Total Sugars 8g, Protein 14g

16. Smoked Salmon and Avocado Salad with Caper Dressing

 **Preparation: 15 minutes**

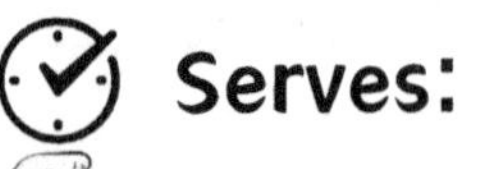 **Total Time: 15 minutes**

Serves: 4

5 oz mixed greens
- 4 oz smoked salmon, flaked
- 1 avocado, diced
- 1/4 cup thinly sliced red onion
- 2 tbsp capers, drained and chopped

Caper Dressing:
- 2 tbsp olive oil
- 2 tbsp lemon juice
- 1 tbsp Dijon mustard
- 1 tbsp chopped capers
- 1 garlic clove, minced
- Salt and pepper to taste

1. In a large salad bowl, combine the mixed greens, flaked smoked salmon, diced avocado, and sliced red onion.

2. In a small bowl, whisk together the ingredients for the caper dressing.

3. Drizzle the caper dressing over the salad and toss gently to coat.

4. Sprinkle the chopped capers over the top of the salad.

5. Serve the smoked salmon and avocado salad immediately.

Nutrition Facts: Calories 260, Total Fat 19g, Saturated Fat 3g, Cholesterol 30mg, Sodium 580mg, Total Carbohydrates 9g, Dietary Fiber 5g, Total Sugars 2g, Protein 15g

 **Preparation: 20 minutes**

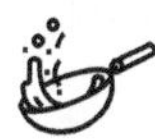 **Cook Time: 15 minutes**

 **Total Time: 35 minutes**

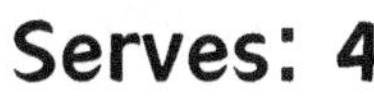 **Serves: 4**

1 cup cooked quinoa
- 1 lb boneless, skinless chicken breasts, grilled and diced
- 1 cup diced cucumber
- 1/2 cup diced red bell pepper
- 1/4 cup crumbled feta cheese
- 2 tbsp chopped fresh parsley

Pomegranate Dressing:
- 1/4 cup pomegranate juice
- 2 tbsp olive oil
- 1 tbsp red wine vinegar
- 1 tsp Dijon mustard
- 1 garlic clove, minced
- Salt and pepper to taste

17. Chicken and Quinoa Salad with Pomegranate Dressing

1. In a large salad bowl, combine the cooked quinoa, grilled and diced chicken, diced cucumber, diced red bell pepper, crumbled feta cheese, and chopped parsley.

2. In a small bowl, whisk together the ingredients for the pomegranate dressing. Season with salt and pepper to taste.

3. Drizzle the pomegranate dressing over the salad and toss gently to coat.

4. Serve the chicken and quinoa salad immediately.

Nutrition Facts: Calories 330, Total Fat 13g, Saturated Fat 3g, Cholesterol 70mg, Sodium 350mg, Total Carbohydrates 22g, Dietary Fiber 4g, Total Sugars 7g, Protein 32g

18. Turkey Bacon and Spinach Salad with Mustard Vinaigrette

 **Preparation: 15 minutes**

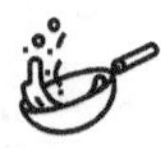 **Cook Time: 10 minutes**

 **Total Time: 25 minutes**

 **Serves: 4**

6 oz baby spinach
- 4 slices turkey bacon, cooked and crumbled
- 1 hard-boiled egg, chopped
- 1/2 cup cherry tomatoes, halved
- 1/4 cup sliced cucumber
- 2 tbsp shredded carrots
- 2 tbsp crumbled feta cheese

Mustard Vinaigrette:
- 2 tbsp red wine vinegar
- 1 tbsp Dijon mustard
- 1 tbsp olive oil
- 1 tsp honey
- 1 garlic clove, minced
- Salt and pepper to taste

1. In a large salad bowl, combine the baby spinach, crumbled turkey bacon, chopped hard-boiled egg, cherry tomatoes, sliced cucumber, and shredded carrots.

2. In a small bowl, whisk together the ingredients for the mustard vinaigrette. Season with salt and pepper to taste.

3. Drizzle the mustard vinaigrette over the salad and toss gently to coat.

4. Sprinkle the crumbled feta cheese over the top of the salad.

5. Serve the turkey bacon and spinach salad immediately.

Nutrition Facts: Calories 180, Total Fat 12g, Saturated Fat 3g, Cholesterol 95mg, Sodium 450mg, Total Carbohydrates 8g, Dietary Fiber 2g, Total Sugars 4g, Protein 12g

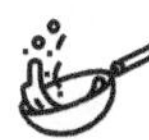 **Preparation: 20 minutes**

 **Cook Time: 30 minutes**

Total Time: 50 minutes

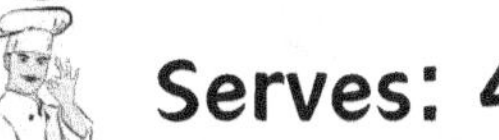 **Serves: 4**

 1 cup cooked wild rice
- 1 lb boneless, skinless chicken breasts, grilled and diced
- 1/2 cup dried cranberries
- 1/2 cup chopped walnuts
- 1/4 cup diced celery
- 2 tbsp chopped green onions
- 2 tbsp chopped parsley

Dressing:
- 2 tbsp olive oil
- 2 tbsp apple cider vinegar
- 1 tbsp Dijon mustard
- 1 tsp honey
- 1 garlic clove, minced
- Salt and pepper to taste

19. Wild Rice and Chicken Salad with Cranberries and Walnuts

1. In a large bowl, combine the cooked wild rice, grilled and diced chicken, dried cranberries, chopped walnuts, diced celery, green onions, and chopped parsley.

2. In a small bowl, whisk together the ingredients for the dressing. Season with salt and pepper to taste.

3. Drizzle the dressing over the wild rice and chicken salad and toss gently to coat.

4. Serve the salad chilled or at room temperature.

Nutrition Facts: Calories 380, Total Fat 18g, Saturated Fat 2g, Cholesterol 70mg, Sodium 220mg, Total Carbohydrates 28g, Dietary Fiber 4g, Total Sugars 12g, Protein 29g

🕐 **Preparation: 15 minutes**

Cook Time: 10 minutes

Total Time: 25 minutes

Serves: 4

- 8 oz ground bison
- 5 oz baby arugula
- 1 cup blueberries
- 1/4 cup crumbled feta cheese
- 2 tbsp toasted sliced almonds

Blueberry Dressing:
- 1/2 cup fresh blueberries
- 2 tbsp balsamic vinegar
- 1 tbsp olive oil
- 1 tsp honey
- 1 garlic clove, minced
- Salt and pepper to taste

20. Bison and Arugula Salad with Blueberry Dressing

1. In a skillet over medium-high heat, cook the ground bison until browned and cooked through, 5-7 minutes. Drain any excess fat and let the bison cool slightly.

2. In a large salad bowl, combine the baby arugula, cooked bison, fresh blueberries, crumbled feta cheese, and toasted sliced almonds.

3. In a blender or food processor, blend the ingredients for the blueberry dressing until smooth.

4. Drizzle the blueberry dressing over the salad and toss gently to coat.

5. Serve the bison and arugula salad immediately.

Nutrition Facts: Calories 260, Total Fat 15g, Saturated Fat 4g, Cholesterol 55mg, Sodium 320mg, Total Carbohydrates 14g, Dietary Fiber 4g, Total Sugars 9g, Protein 20g

Preparation: 15 minutes

Total Time: 15 minutes

Serves: 4

- 1 cup cooked quinoa
- 2 cups shredded rainbow carrots
- 1/2 cup diced cucumber
- 1/4 cup chopped fresh parsley
- 2 tbsp toasted pumpkin seeds

Lemon-Tahini Dressing:
- 2 tbsp tahini
- 2 tbsp lemon juice
- 1 tbsp olive oil
- 1 garlic clove, minced
- 1 tsp honey
- Salt and pepper to taste

1. Rainbow Carrot and Quinoa Salad with Lemon-Tahini Dressing

1. In a large salad bowl, combine the cooked quinoa, shredded rainbow carrots, diced cucumber, and chopped parsley.

2. In a small bowl, whisk together the ingredients for the lemon-tahini dressing. Season with salt and pepper to taste.

3. Drizzle the lemon-tahini dressing over the salad and toss gently to coat.

4. Sprinkle the toasted pumpkin seeds over the top of the salad.

5. Serve the rainbow carrot and quinoa salad immediately.

Nutrition Facts: Calories 220, Total Fat 11g, Saturated Fat 1.5g, Cholesterol 0mg, Sodium 120mg, Total Carbohydrates 25g, Dietary Fiber 5g, Total Sugars 6g, Protein 7g

 **Preparation: 15 minutes**

 **Total Time: 15 minutes**

Serves: 4

- 2 bell peppers (any color), sliced
- 1 cucumber, sliced
- 1/2 red onion, thinly sliced
- 1/4 cup chopped fresh herbs (such as parsley, basil, and dill)

Herb Vinaigrette:
- 2 tbsp red wine vinegar
- 1 tbsp olive oil
- 1 tbsp Dijon mustard
- 1 garlic clove, minced
- 1 tsp honey
- Salt and pepper to taste

2. Bell Pepper and Cucumber Salad with Herb Vinaigrette

1. In a large salad bowl, combine the sliced bell peppers, sliced cucumber, and thinly sliced red onion.

2. In a small bowl, whisk together the ingredients for the herb vinaigrette. Season with salt and pepper to taste.

3. Drizzle the herb vinaigrette over the salad and toss gently to coat.

4. Sprinkle the chopped fresh herbs over the top of the salad.

5. Serve the bell pepper and cucumber salad immediately.

Nutrition Facts: Calories 90, Total Fat 5g, Saturated Fat 0.5g, Cholesterol 0mg, Sodium 150mg, Total Carbohydrates 10g, Dietary Fiber 2g, Total Sugars 6g, Protein 2g

3. Roasted Veggie Salad with Sweet Potato, Beet, and Carrot

 **Preparation: 20 minutes**

 **Cook Time: 30 minutes**

 **Total Time: 50 minutes**

Serves: 4

- 1 medium sweet potato, peeled and diced
- 2 medium beets, peeled and diced
- 2 carrots, peeled and diced
- 2 tbsp olive oil
- Salt and pepper to taste
- 5 oz mixed greens
- 1/4 cup crumbled feta cheese
- 2 tbsp toasted pumpkin seeds

Balsamic Vinaigrette:
- 2 tbsp balsamic vinegar
- 1 tbsp olive oil
- 1 tsp Dijon mustard
- 1 tsp honey
- 1 garlic clove, minced
- Salt and pepper to taste

1. Preheat the oven to 400°F. Line a baking sheet with parchment paper.

2. In a large bowl, toss the diced sweet potato, beets, and carrots with the olive oil. Season with salt and pepper.

3. Spread the vegetables in a single layer on the prepared baking sheet. Roast for 25-30 minutes, stirring halfway, until the vegetables are tender and lightly browned.

4. Allow the roasted vegetables to cool slightly.

5. In a large salad bowl, combine the mixed greens, roasted vegetables, crumbled feta cheese, and toasted pumpkin seeds.

6. In a small bowl, whisk together the ingredients for the balsamic vinaigrette. Season with salt and pepper to taste.

7. Drizzle the balsamic vinaigrette over the salad and toss gently to coat.

8. Serve the roasted veggie salad warm or at room temperature.

Nutrition Facts: Calories 250, Total Fat 14g, Saturated Fat 3g, Cholesterol 10mg, Sodium 320mg, Total Carbohydrates 25g, Dietary Fiber 6g, Total Sugars 10g, Protein 7g

 **Preparation: 15 minutes**

 **Total Time: 15 minutes**

 **Serves: 4**

- 2 cups cherry tomatoes, halved
- 1 cucumber, sliced
- 1/2 red onion, thinly sliced
- 1/4 cup crumbled feta cheese
- 2 tbsp chopped fresh basil

Dressing:
- 2 tbsp olive oil
- 1 tbsp red wine vinegar
- 1 tsp Dijon mustard
- 1 garlic clove, minced
- Salt and pepper to taste

4. Tomato, Cucumber, and Red Onion Salad with Feta

1. In a large salad bowl, combine the halved cherry tomatoes, sliced cucumber, thinly sliced red onion, crumbled feta cheese, and chopped fresh basil.

2. In a small bowl, whisk together the ingredients for the dressing. Season with salt and pepper to taste.

3. Drizzle the dressing over the salad and toss gently to coat.

4. Serve the tomato, cucumber, and red onion salad immediately.

Nutrition Facts: Calories 120, Total Fat 8g, Saturated Fat 2g, Cholesterol 10mg, Sodium 220mg, Total Carbohydrates 10g, Dietary Fiber 2g, Total Sugars 6g, Protein 4g

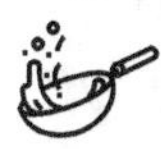
Preparation: 20 minutes

Cook Time: 15 minutes

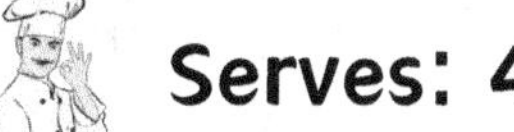
Total Time: 35 minutes

Serves: 4

- 1 zucchini, sliced
- 1 yellow squash, sliced
- 1 red bell pepper, sliced
- 1 red onion, sliced
- 2 tbsp olive oil
- Salt and pepper to taste
- 5 oz mixed greens
- 2 tbsp crumbled feta cheese
- 2 tbsp toasted pine nuts

Balsamic Reduction:
- 1/2 cup balsamic vinegar
- 1 tsp honey

5. Grilled Vegetable Salad with Balsamic Reduction

1. Preheat a grill or grill pan to medium-high heat.

2. In a large bowl, toss the sliced zucchini, yellow squash, red bell pepper, and red onion with the olive oil. Season with salt and pepper.

3. Grill the vegetables for 2-3 minutes per side, or until they are tender and have grill marks.

4. In a small saucepan, combine the balsamic vinegar and honey. Bring to a simmer and cook for 5-7 minutes, or until the mixture has reduced by half and thickened slightly.

5. In a large salad bowl, arrange the mixed greens. Top with the grilled vegetables, crumbled feta cheese, and toasted pine nuts.

6. Drizzle the balsamic reduction over the salad.

7. Serve the grilled vegetable salad immediately.

Nutrition Facts: Calories 180, Total Fat 12g, Saturated Fat 3g, Cholesterol 10mg, Sodium 220mg, Total Carbohydrates 15g, Dietary Fiber 3g, Total Sugars 9g, Protein 5g

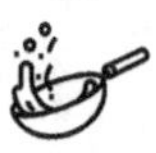

Preparation: 20 minutes

Total Time: 20 minutes

Serves: 4

- 3 cups riced cauliflower
- 1 cup diced cucumber
- 1/2 cup diced red bell pepper
- 1/2 cup diced red onion
- 1/4 cup chopped fresh parsley
- 2 tbsp chopped fresh mint
- 2 tbsp toasted sliced almonds

Dressing:
- 2 tbsp olive oil
- 2 tbsp lemon juice
- 1 tbsp Dijon mustard
- 1 tsp honey
- 1 garlic clove, minced
- Salt and pepper to taste

6. Cauliflower Rice Salad with Mixed Veggies

1. In a large salad bowl, combine the riced cauliflower, diced cucumber, diced red bell pepper, diced red onion, chopped parsley, and chopped mint.

2. In a small bowl, whisk together the ingredients for the dressing. Season with salt and pepper to taste.

3. Drizzle the dressing over the cauliflower rice salad and toss gently to coat.

4. Sprinkle the toasted sliced almonds over the top of the salad.

5. Serve the cauliflower rice salad immediately.

Nutrition Facts: Calories 150, Total Fat 10g, Saturated Fat 1g, Cholesterol 0mg, Sodium 180mg, Total Carbohydrates 12g, Dietary Fiber 4g, Total Sugars 5g, Protein 4g

Preparation: 15 minutes

Total Time: 15 minutes

Serves: 4

- 2 medium zucchini, sliced
- 1 pint cherry tomatoes, halved
- 1/4 cup fresh basil leaves, chopped
- 2 tbsp pine nuts, toasted
- 2 tbsp grated Parmesan cheese

Basil Pesto:
- 2 cups fresh basil leaves
- 2 tbsp pine nuts
- 1 garlic clove
- 2 tbsp olive oil
- 1 tbsp lemon juice
- Salt and pepper to taste

7. Zucchini and Tomato Salad with Basil Pesto

1. In a large salad bowl, combine the sliced zucchini, halved cherry tomatoes, chopped fresh basil, toasted pine nuts, and grated Parmesan cheese.

2. In a food processor or blender, blend the ingredients for the basil pesto until smooth.

3. Drizzle the basil pesto over the zucchini and tomato salad and toss gently to coat.

4. Serve the zucchini and tomato salad immediately.

Nutrition Facts: Calories 160, Total Fat 13g, Saturated Fat 2g, Cholesterol 5mg, Sodium 120mg, Total Carbohydrates 8g, Dietary Fiber 3g, Total Sugars 4g, Protein 5g

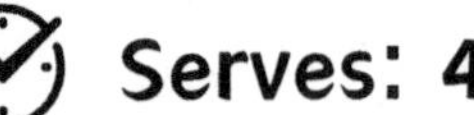

8. Sweet Corn and Black Bean Salad with Lime Vinaigrette

🕐 **Preparation: 15 minutes**

Total Time: 15 minutes

Serves: 4

- 2 cups cooked sweet corn kernels
- 1 (15 oz) can black beans, drained and rinsed
- 1 cup diced tomatoes
- 1/2 cup diced red onion
- 1/4 cup chopped fresh cilantro
- 2 tbsp chopped jalapeño (optional)

Lime Vinaigrette:
- 2 tbsp lime juice
- 1 tbsp olive oil
- 1 tsp honey
- 1 garlic clove, minced
- 1/4 tsp ground cumin
- Salt and pepper to taste

1. In a large salad bowl, combine the cooked sweet corn kernels, drained and rinsed black beans, diced tomatoes, diced red onion, chopped cilantro, and chopped jalapeño (if using).

2. In a small bowl, whisk together the ingredients for the lime vinaigrette. Season with salt and pepper to taste.

3. Drizzle the lime vinaigrette over the sweet corn and black bean salad and toss gently to coat.

4. Serve the salad immediately or chill in the refrigerator until ready to serve.

Nutrition Facts: Calories 180, Total Fat 6g, Saturated Fat 1g, Cholesterol 0mg, Sodium 320mg, Total Carbohydrates 27g, Dietary Fiber 7g, Total Sugars 6g, Protein 7g

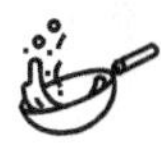

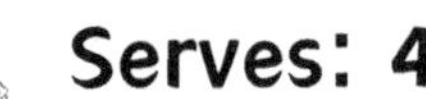

Preparation: 20 minutes

Cook Time: 25 minutes

Total Time: 45 minutes

Serves: 4

- 1 small butternut squash, peeled, seeded, and cubed
- 2 tbsp olive oil
- Salt and pepper to taste
- 4 cups chopped kale
- 1/4 cup dried cranberries
- 1/4 cup toasted pumpkin seeds
- 2 tbsp crumbled feta cheese

Maple Balsamic Vinaigrette:
- 2 tbsp balsamic vinegar
- 1 tbsp maple syrup
- 1 tbsp olive oil
- 1 tsp Dijon mustard
- 1 garlic clove, minced
- Salt and pepper to taste

9. Roasted Butternut Squash and Kale Salad

1. Preheat the oven to 400°F. Line a baking sheet with parchment paper.

2. Toss the cubed butternut squash with 2 tbsp of olive oil. Season with salt and pepper.

3. Roast the butternut squash for 20-25 minutes, or until tender and lightly browned. Allow to cool slightly.

4. In a large salad bowl, combine the roasted butternut squash, chopped kale, dried cranberries, toasted pumpkin seeds, and crumbled feta cheese.

5. In a small bowl, whisk together the ingredients for the maple balsamic vinaigrette. Season with salt and pepper to taste.

6. Drizzle the vinaigrette over the salad and toss gently to coat.

7. Serve the roasted butternut squash and kale salad immediately.

Nutrition Facts: Calories 260, Total Fat 13g, Saturated Fat 3g, Cholesterol 10mg, Sodium 220mg, Total Carbohydrates 32g, Dietary Fiber 6g, Total Sugars 12g, Protein 7g

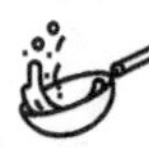

Preparation: 15 minutes

Total Time: 15 minutes

Serves: 4

- 1 cup thinly sliced radishes
- 1 cup julienned jicama
- 1/4 cup chopped fresh cilantro
- 2 tbsp chopped green onions

Cilantro Dressing:
- 1/4 cup olive oil
- 2 tbsp lime juice
- 2 tbsp chopped fresh cilantro
- 1 garlic clove, minced
- 1 tsp honey
- Salt and pepper to taste

10. Radish and Jicama Salad with Cilantro Dressing

1. In a large salad bowl, combine the thinly sliced radishes, julienned jicama, chopped cilantro, and chopped green onions.

2. In a small bowl, whisk together the ingredients for the cilantro dressing. Season with salt and pepper to taste.

3. Drizzle the cilantro dressing over the radish and jicama salad and toss gently to coat.

4. Serve the salad immediately.

Nutrition Facts: Calories 120, Total Fat 9g, Saturated Fat 1g, Cholesterol 0mg, Sodium 120mg, Total Carbohydrates 10g, Dietary Fiber 3g, Total Sugars 4g, Protein 1g

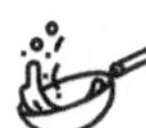 **Preparation: 15 minutes**

 **Cook Time: 10 minutes**

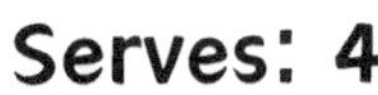 **Total Time: 25 minutes**

Serves: 4

- 1 lb asparagus, trimmed
- 1 red bell pepper, sliced
- 2 tbsp olive oil
- Salt and pepper to taste
- 5 oz mixed greens
- 2 tbsp crumbled feta cheese
- 2 tbsp toasted pine nuts

Lemon Vinaigrette:
- 2 tbsp lemon juice
- 1 tbsp olive oil
- 1 tsp Dijon mustard
- 1 garlic clove, minced
- Salt and pepper to taste

11. Grilled Asparagus and Red Pepper Salad

1. Preheat a grill or grill pan to medium-high heat.

2. In a large bowl, toss the asparagus and red bell pepper slices with 2 tbsp of olive oil. Season with salt and pepper.

3. Grill the asparagus and red pepper for 2-3 minutes per side, or until they are tender and have grill marks.

4. In a large salad bowl, arrange the mixed greens. Top with the grilled asparagus and red pepper slices.

5. Sprinkle the crumbled feta cheese and toasted pine nuts over the salad.

6. In a small bowl, whisk together the ingredients for the lemon vinaigrette. Season with salt and pepper to taste.

7. Drizzle the lemon vinaigrette over the salad and toss gently to coat.

8. Serve the grilled asparagus and red pepper salad immediately.

Nutrition Facts: Calories 180, Total Fat 14g, Saturated Fat 3g, Cholesterol 10mg, Sodium 220mg, Total Carbohydrates 10g, Dietary Fiber 4g, Total Sugars 4g, Protein 6g

🕐 **Preparation: 20 minutes**

🍳 **Cook Time: 20 minutes**

✓ **Total Time: 40 minutes**

👨‍🍳 **Serves: 4**

- 1 lb Brussels sprouts, trimmed and halved
- 2 tbsp olive oil
- Salt and pepper to taste
- 4 oz mixed greens
- 1/2 cup pomegranate arils
- 1/4 cup toasted sliced almonds
- 2 tbsp crumbled feta cheese

Balsamic Vinaigrette:
- 2 tbsp balsamic vinegar
- 1 tbsp olive oil
- 1 tsp Dijon mustard
- 1 tsp honey
- 1 garlic clove, minced
- Salt and pepper to taste

12. Roasted Brussels Sprouts and Pomegranate Salad

1. Preheat the oven to 400°F. Line a baking sheet with parchment paper.

2. Toss the halved Brussels sprouts with 2 tbsp of olive oil. Season with salt and pepper.

3. Roast the Brussels sprouts for 18-20 minutes, or until they are tender and lightly browned. Allow to cool slightly.

4. In a large salad bowl, combine the roasted Brussels sprouts, mixed greens, pomegranate arils, toasted sliced almonds, and crumbled feta cheese.

5. In a small bowl, whisk together the ingredients for the balsamic vinaigrette. Season with salt and pepper to taste.

6. Drizzle the balsamic vinaigrette over the salad and toss gently to coat.

7. Serve the roasted Brussels sprouts and pomegranate salad immediately.

Nutrition Facts: Calories 220, Total Fat 14g, Saturated Fat 3g, Cholesterol 10mg, Sodium 220mg, Total Carbohydrates 20g, Dietary Fiber 6g, Total Sugars 8g, Protein 7g

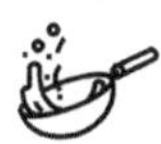

Preparation: 20 minutes

Total Time: 20 minutes

Serves: 4

- 1 (15 oz) can mixed beans, drained and rinsed
- 1 cup diced cucumber
- 1/2 cup diced tomatoes
- 1/4 cup diced red onion
- 1/4 cup chopped fresh mint
- 2 tbsp chopped fresh parsley

Mint Dressing:
- 1/4 cup olive oil
- 2 tbsp white wine vinegar
- 2 tbsp chopped fresh mint
- 1 garlic clove, minced
- 1 tsp honey
- Salt and pepper to taste

13. Mixed Bean and Veggie Salad with Mint Dressing

1. In a large salad bowl, combine the drained and rinsed mixed beans, diced cucumber, diced tomatoes, diced red onion, chopped fresh mint, and chopped fresh parsley.

2. In a small bowl, whisk together the ingredients for the mint dressing. Season with salt and pepper to taste.

3. Drizzle the mint dressing over the mixed bean and veggie salad and toss gently to coat.

4. Serve the salad immediately or chill in the refrigerator until ready to serve.

Nutrition Facts: Calories 180, Total Fat 10g, Saturated Fat 1.5g, Cholesterol 0mg, Sodium 280mg, Total Carbohydrates 18g, Dietary Fiber 5g, Total Sugars 4g, Protein 6g

Preparation: 15 minutes

Total Time: 15 minutes

Serves: 4

- 2 cups shredded green cabbage
- 1 cup shredded carrots
- 1/2 cup diced red bell pepper
- 1/4 cup chopped fresh cilantro
- 2 tbsp chopped green onions

Dressing:
- 2 tbsp apple cider vinegar
- 1 tbsp olive oil
- 1 tsp Dijon mustard
- 1 tsp honey
- Salt and pepper to taste

14. Cabbage, Carrot, and Bell Pepper Slaw

1. In a large salad bowl, combine the shredded green cabbage, shredded carrots, diced red bell pepper, chopped cilantro, and chopped green onions.

2. In a small bowl, whisk together the ingredients for the dressing. Season with salt and pepper to taste.

3. Drizzle the dressing over the cabbage, carrot, and bell pepper slaw and toss gently to coat.

4. Serve the slaw immediately or chill in the refrigerator until ready to serve.

Nutrition Facts: Calories 90, Total Fat 5g, Saturated Fat 0.5g, Cholesterol 0mg, Sodium 150mg, Total Carbohydrates 11g, Dietary Fiber 3g, Total Sugars 6g, Protein 2g

Preparation: 20 minutes

Cook Time: 30 minutes

Total Time: 50 minutes

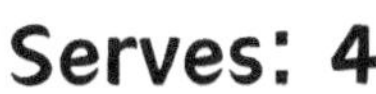

Serves: 4

- 3 medium beets, peeled and cubed
- 3 medium carrots, peeled and cubed
- 2 tbsp olive oil
- Salt and pepper to taste
- 5 oz mixed greens
- 2 tbsp toasted pumpkin seeds
- 2 tbsp crumbled feta cheese

Tahini Dressing:
- 2 tbsp tahini
- 2 tbsp lemon juice
- 1 tbsp water
- 1 garlic clove, minced
- 1 tsp honey
- Salt and pepper to taste

15. Roasted Beet and Carrot Salad with Tahini Dressing

1. Preheat the oven to 400°F. Line a baking sheet with parchment paper.

2. Toss the cubed beets and carrots with 2 tbsp of olive oil. Season with salt and pepper.

3. Roast the vegetables for 25-30 minutes, or until they are tender and lightly browned. Allow to cool slightly.

4. In a large salad bowl, arrange the mixed greens. Top with the roasted beets and carrots.

5. Sprinkle the toasted pumpkin seeds and crumbled feta cheese over the salad.

6. In a small bowl, whisk together the ingredients for the tahini dressing. Season with salt and pepper to taste.

7. Drizzle the tahini dressing over the salad and toss gently to coat.

8. Serve the roasted beet and carrot salad immediately.

Nutrition Facts: Calories 220, Total Fat 14g, Saturated Fat 3g, Cholesterol 10mg, Sodium 320mg, Total Carbohydrates 20g, Dietary Fiber 6g, Total Sugars 10g, Protein 6g

🕐 **Preparation: 15 minutes**

🥄 **Cook Time: 5 minutes**

✔ **Total Time: 20 minutes**

👨‍🍳 **Serves: 4**

- 1 lb green beans, trimmed and cut into 1-inch pieces
- 1 pint cherry tomatoes, halved
- 1/4 cup chopped fresh basil
- 2 tbsp chopped red onion
- 2 tbsp toasted sliced almonds

Dressing:
- 2 tbsp olive oil
- 1 tbsp balsamic vinegar
- 1 tsp Dijon mustard
- 1 garlic clove, minced
- Salt and pepper to taste

16. Green Bean and Cherry Tomato Salad

1. Bring a medium pot of salted water to a boil. Add the green bean pieces and cook for 3-5 minutes, until tender-crisp. Drain and rinse with cold water to stop the cooking.

2. In a large salad bowl, combine the cooked green beans, halved cherry tomatoes, chopped basil, and chopped red onion.

3. In a small bowl, whisk together the ingredients for the dressing. Season with salt and pepper to taste.

4. Drizzle the dressing over the green bean and tomato salad and toss gently to coat.

5. Sprinkle the toasted sliced almonds over the top of the salad.

6. Serve the green bean and cherry tomato salad immediately.

Nutrition Facts: Calories 130, Total Fat 9g, Saturated Fat 1g, Cholesterol 0mg, Sodium 120mg, Total Carbohydrates 11g, Dietary Fiber 4g, Total Sugars 5g, Protein 3g

Preparation: 15 minutes

Total Time: 15 minutes

Serves: 4

- 2 medium zucchinis, spiralized
- 2 medium carrots, spiralized
- 1/4 cup chopped fresh cilantro
- 2 tbsp chopped green onions

Ginger Dressing:
- 2 tbsp rice vinegar
- 1 tbsp sesame oil
- 1 tbsp grated fresh ginger
- 1 tsp honey
- 1 garlic clove, minced
- Salt and pepper to taste

17. Spiralized Zucchini and Carrot Salad with Ginger Dressing

1. In a large salad bowl, combine the spiralized zucchini, spiralized carrots, chopped cilantro, and chopped green onions.

2. In a small bowl, whisk together the ingredients for the ginger dressing. Season with salt and pepper to taste.

3. Drizzle the ginger dressing over the spiralized zucchini and carrot salad and toss gently to coat.

4. Serve the salad immediately.

Nutrition Facts: Calories 90, Total Fat 5g, Saturated Fat 1g, Cholesterol 0mg, Sodium 120mg, Total Carbohydrates 10g, Dietary Fiber 2g, Total Sugars 5g, Protein 2g

18. Sweet Potato and Spinach Salad with Maple Vinaigrette

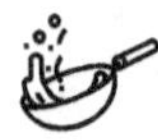 **Preparation: 20 minutes**

 **Cook Time: 20 minutes**

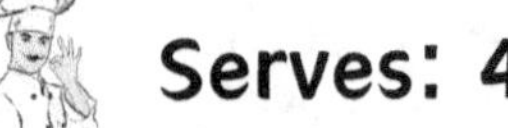 **Total Time: 40 minutes**

Serves: 4

- 2 medium sweet potatoes, peeled and cubed
- 2 tbsp olive oil
- Salt and pepper to taste
- 5 oz baby spinach
- 1/4 cup dried cranberries
- 2 tbsp chopped pecans
- 2 tbsp crumbled feta cheese

Maple Vinaigrette:
- 2 tbsp maple syrup
- 1 tbsp apple cider vinegar
- 1 tbsp olive oil
- 1 tsp Dijon mustard
- 1 garlic clove, minced
- Salt and pepper to taste

1. Preheat the oven to 400°F. Line a baking sheet with parchment paper.

2. Toss the cubed sweet potatoes with 2 tbsp of olive oil. Season with salt and pepper.

3. Roast the sweet potatoes for 18-20 minutes, or until they are tender and lightly browned. Allow to cool slightly.

4. In a large salad bowl, combine the roasted sweet potatoes, baby spinach, dried cranberries, chopped pecans, and crumbled feta cheese.

5. In a small bowl, whisk together the ingredients for the maple vinaigrette. Season with salt and pepper to taste.

6. Drizzle the maple vinaigrette over the salad and toss gently to coat.

7. Serve the sweet potato and spinach salad immediately.

Nutrition Facts: Calories 240, Total Fat 12g, Saturated Fat 3g, Cholesterol 10mg, Sodium 260mg, Total Carbohydrates 30g, Dietary Fiber 5g, Total Sugars 14g, Protein 5g

 **Preparation: 15 minutes**

 **Total Time: 15 minutes**

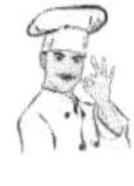 **Serves: 4**

- 2 medium kohlrabi, peeled and julienned
- 1 Granny Smith apple, julienned
- 1/4 cup chopped fresh parsley
- 2 tbsp chopped toasted walnuts

Lemon Dressing:
- 2 tbsp lemon juice
- 1 tbsp olive oil
- 1 tsp Dijon mustard
- 1 tsp honey
- 1 garlic clove, minced
- Salt and pepper to taste

19. Kohlrabi and Apple Salad with Lemon Dressing

1. In a large salad bowl, combine the julienned kohlrabi, julienned Granny Smith apple, chopped parsley, and chopped toasted walnuts.

2. In a small bowl, whisk together the ingredients for the lemon dressing. Season with salt and pepper to taste.

3. Drizzle the lemon dressing over the kohlrabi and apple salad and toss gently to coat.

4. Serve the salad immediately.

Nutrition Facts: Calories 110, Total Fat 6g, Saturated Fat 1g, Cholesterol 0mg, Sodium 120mg, Total Carbohydrates 13g, Dietary Fiber 4g, Total Sugars 7g, Protein 3g

🕐 **Preparation: 20 minutes**

🥣 **Cook Time: 15 minutes**

✓ **Total Time: 35 minutes**

👨‍🍳 **Serves: 4**

- 1 medium eggplant, sliced into 1/2-inch rounds
- 2 tbsp olive oil, plus more for brushing
- Salt and pepper to taste
- 1 pint cherry tomatoes, halved
- 1/4 cup chopped fresh basil
- 2 tbsp balsamic glaze

20. Grilled Eggplant and Tomato Salad with Balsamic Glaze

1. Preheat a grill or grill pan to medium-high heat.

2. Brush the eggplant slices with olive oil on both sides and season with salt and pepper.

3. Grill the eggplant slices for 3-4 minutes per side, or until they are tender and have grill marks. Transfer to a plate and let cool slightly.

4. In a large salad bowl, combine the grilled eggplant slices, halved cherry tomatoes, and chopped fresh basil.

5. Drizzle the balsamic glaze over the salad and toss gently to coat.

6. Serve the grilled eggplant and tomato salad immediately.

Nutrition Facts: Calories 120, Total Fat 8g, Saturated Fat 1g, Cholesterol 0mg, Sodium 150mg, Total Carbohydrates 12g, Dietary Fiber 4g, Total Sugars 7g, Protein 2g

🕐 **Preparation: 10 minutes**

Cook Time: 0 minutes

Total Time: 10 minutes

Serves: 4

- 5 oz baby arugula
- 8 fresh figs, quartered
- 1/2 cup toasted walnuts
- 2 tbsp balsamic vinegar
- 1 tbsp extra-virgin olive oil
- 1/4 tsp sea salt
- 1/4 tsp freshly ground black pepper

1. Arugula and Fig Salad with Walnuts

1. In a large bowl, combine the arugula, figs, and walnuts.

2. Drizzle the balsamic vinegar and olive oil over the salad, and season with salt and pepper.

3. Toss gently to coat.

Nutrition Facts: 150 calories | 10g fat | 15g carbs | 4g fiber | 3g protein

 **Preparation: 10 minutes**

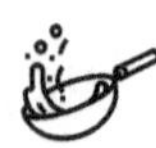 **Cook Time: 5 minutes**

 **Total Time: 15 minutes**

 **Serves: 4**

- 6 cups mixed greens (spinach, arugula, baby kale)
- 1 medium apple, cored and thinly sliced
- 1/2 cup toasted walnuts
- 1/4 cup crumbled blue cheese
- 2 tbsp olive oil
- 1 tbsp apple cider vinegar
- 1 tsp Dijon mustard
- 1 tsp honey
- Salt and pepper to taste

2. Mixed Greens with Apple, Walnut, and Blue Cheese

1. In a large salad bowl, combine the mixed greens, apple slices, toasted walnuts, and crumbled blue cheese.

2. In a small bowl, whisk together the olive oil, apple cider vinegar, Dijon mustard, and honey. Season with salt and pepper to taste.

3. Drizzle the dressing over the salad and toss gently to coat.

4. Serve immediately.

Nutrition Facts: 210 calories, 16g fat, 4g saturated fat, 10mg cholesterol, 220mg sodium, 16g carbohydrates, 4g fiber, 10g sugar, 5g protein.

This anti-inflammatory salad is packed with nutrient-rich greens, heart-healthy walnuts, and tangy blue cheese, making it a delicious and wholesome option.

 **Preparation: 10 minutes**

 **Cook Time: 0 minutes**

Total Time: 10 minutes

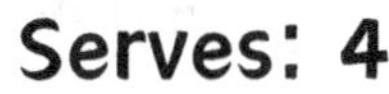 **Serves: 4**

- 5 cups fresh spinach leaves
- 1 cup fresh strawberries, sliced
- 1/4 cup sliced almonds, toasted
- 2 tbsp balsamic vinegar
- 1 tbsp olive oil
- 1 tsp Dijon mustard
- 1 tsp honey
- Salt and pepper to taste

3. Strawberry and Spinach Salad with Almonds

1. In a large salad bowl, combine the spinach leaves, sliced strawberries, and toasted almonds.
2. In a small bowl, whisk together the balsamic vinegar, olive oil, Dijon mustard, and honey. Season with salt and pepper to taste.
3. Drizzle the dressing over the salad and toss gently to coat.
4. Serve immediately.

Nutrition Facts: 120 calories, 8g fat, 1g saturated fat, 0mg cholesterol, 150mg sodium, 10g carbohydrates, 3g fiber, 6g sugar, 3g protein.

This refreshing and anti-inflammatory salad features nutrient-rich spinach, sweet strawberries, and crunchy almonds. The balsamic vinaigrette adds a tangy and slightly sweet flavor to the dish.

 **Preparation: 10 minutes**

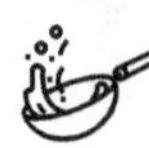 **Cook Time: 5 minutes**

 **Total Time: 15 minutes**

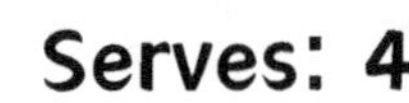 **Serves: 4**

- 6 cups mixed greens (such as spinach, arugula, and baby kale)
- 2 ripe pears, cored and sliced
- 1/2 cup toasted pecans
- 2 tbsp olive oil
- 1 tbsp apple cider vinegar
- 1 tbsp pure maple syrup
- 1 tsp Dijon mustard
- Salt and pepper to taste

4. Pear and Pecan Salad with Maple Vinaigrette

1. In a large salad bowl, combine the mixed greens, sliced pears, and toasted pecans.

2. In a small bowl, whisk together the olive oil, apple cider vinegar, maple syrup, and Dijon mustard. Season with salt and pepper to taste.

3. Drizzle the maple vinaigrette over the salad and toss gently to coat.

4. Serve immediately.

Nutrition Facts: 190 calories, 14g fat, 2g saturated fat, 0mg cholesterol, 150mg sodium, 16g carbohydrates, 4g fiber, 10g sugar, 3g protein.

This anti-inflammatory salad features sweet pears, crunchy pecans, and a tangy-sweet maple vinaigrette. The combination of flavors and textures makes for a delightful and nourishing meal.

 **Preparation: 15 minutes**

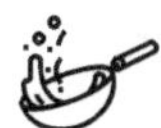 **Cook Time: 0 minutes**

 **Total Time: 15 minutes**

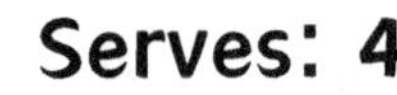 **Serves: 4**

- 5 cups mixed greens (such as spinach, arugula, and baby kale)
- 1 ripe mango, peeled and cubed
- 1 avocado, diced
- 1/4 cup roasted cashews
- 2 tbsp cashew butter
- 2 tbsp water
- 1 tbsp apple cider vinegar
- 1 tsp honey
- 1/4 tsp ground cumin
- Salt and pepper to taste

5. Mango and Avocado Salad with Cashew Dressing

1. In a large salad bowl, combine the mixed greens, mango cubes, and diced avocado.

2. In a small bowl, whisk together the cashew butter, water, apple cider vinegar, honey, and ground cumin. Season with salt and pepper to taste.

3. Drizzle the cashew dressing over the salad and toss gently to coat.

4. Sprinkle the roasted cashews over the top.

5. Serve immediately.

Nutrition Facts: 240 calories, 16g fat, 2.5g saturated fat, 0mg cholesterol, 90mg sodium, 22g carbohydrates, 6g fiber, 14g sugar, 5g protein.

This anti-inflammatory salad features the sweet and creamy flavors of mango and avocado, complemented by the nutty cashew dressing. The crunchy roasted cashews add a delightful texture to the dish.

6. Kale and Pomegranate Salad with Pistachios

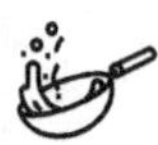 **Preparation: 15 minutes**

 **Cook Time: 0 minutes**

 **Total Time: 15 minutes**

Serves: 4

- 6 cups chopped kale
- 1 cup pomegranate arils
- 1/2 cup roasted and salted pistachios, chopped
- 2 tablespoons olive oil
- 2 tablespoons balsamic vinegar
- 1 tablespoon honey
- 1/4 teaspoon salt
- 1/4 teaspoon black pepper

1. In a large bowl, combine the chopped kale, pomegranate arils, and chopped pistachios.

2. In a small bowl, whisk together the olive oil, balsamic vinegar, honey, salt, and black pepper.

3. Drizzle the dressing over the kale mixture and toss to coat evenly.

4. Serve immediately.

NUTRITION FACTS: Calories 190 | Total Fat 12g | Saturated Fat 2g | Cholesterol 0mg | Sodium 240mg | Total Carbohydrates 19g | Dietary Fiber 4g | Total Sugars 12g | Protein 5g

7. Berry and Mixed Nut Salad with Citrus Dressing

 **Preparation: 20 minutes**

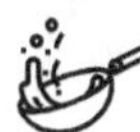 **Cook Time: 0 minutes**

 **Total Time: 20 minutes**

Serves: 4

- 5 cups mixed greens
- 1 cup mixed berries (such as blueberries, raspberries, and blackberries)
- 1/2 cup mixed nuts (such as almonds, walnuts, and pecans), chopped
- 2 tablespoons olive oil
- 2 tablespoons orange juice
- 1 tablespoon lemon juice
- 1 teaspoon honey
- 1/4 teaspoon salt
- 1/4 teaspoon black pepper

1. In a large bowl, combine the mixed greens, mixed berries, and chopped mixed nuts.

2. In a small bowl, whisk together the olive oil, orange juice, lemon juice, honey, salt, and black pepper.

3. Drizzle the dressing over the salad and toss to coat evenly.

4. Serve immediately.

NUTRITION FACTS: Calories 210 | Total Fat 15g | Saturated Fat 2g | Cholesterol 0mg | Sodium 210mg | Total Carbohydrates 18g | Dietary Fiber 5g | Total Sugars 10g | Protein 5g

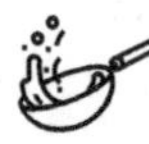 **Preparation: 15 minutes**

 **Cook Time: 0 minutes**

Total Time: 15 minutes

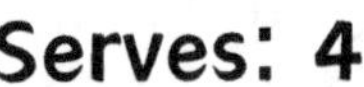 **Serves: 4**

- 6 cups baby spinach
- 1 cup fresh raspberries
- 1/2 cup sliced almonds, toasted
- 2 tablespoons olive oil
- 1 tablespoon balsamic vinegar
- 1 teaspoon Dijon mustard
- 1 teaspoon honey
- 1/4 teaspoon salt
- 1/4 teaspoon black pepper

8. Raspberry and Almond Salad with Spinach

1. In a large bowl, combine the baby spinach, fresh raspberries, and toasted sliced almonds.

2. In a small bowl, whisk together the olive oil, balsamic vinegar, Dijon mustard, honey, salt, and black pepper.

3. Drizzle the dressing over the salad and toss to coat evenly.

4. Serve immediately.

NUTRITION FACTS: Calories 170 | Total Fat 13g | Saturated Fat 2g | Cholesterol 0mg | Sodium 230mg | Total Carbohydrates 12g | Dietary Fiber 5g | Total Sugars 6g | Protein 5g

 **Preparation: 20 minutes**

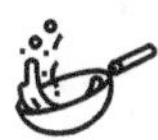 **Cook Time: 0 minutes**

 **Total Time: 20 minutes**

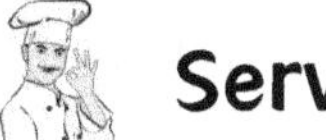 **Serves: 4**

- 6 cups mixed greens
- 2 medium apples, cored and sliced
- 1/2 cup toasted hazelnuts, chopped
- 2 tablespoons apple cider vinegar
- 1 tablespoon olive oil
- 1 teaspoon Dijon mustard
- 1 teaspoon honey
- 1/4 teaspoon salt
- 1/4 teaspoon black pepper

9. Apple and Hazelnut Salad with Cider Vinaigrette

1. In a large bowl, combine the mixed greens, sliced apples, and chopped toasted hazelnuts.

2. In a small bowl, whisk together the apple cider vinegar, olive oil, Dijon mustard, honey, salt, and black pepper.

3. Drizzle the dressing over the salad and toss to coat evenly.

4. Serve immediately.

NUTRITION FACTS: Calories 190 | Total Fat 12g | Saturated Fat 1g | Cholesterol 0mg | Sodium 240mg | Total Carbohydrates 19g | Dietary Fiber 5g | Total Sugars 12g | Protein 4g

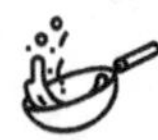 **Preparation: 20 minutes**

 **Cook Time: 0 minutes**

Total Time: 20 minutes

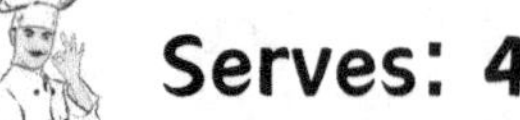 **Serves: 4**

- 4 cups mixed greens
- 2 ruby red grapefruits, peeled and segmented
- 1 avocado, diced
- 1/4 cup toasted pine nuts
- 2 tablespoons olive oil
- 2 tablespoons white wine vinegar
- 1 teaspoon honey
- 1/4 teaspoon salt
- 1/4 teaspoon black pepper

10. Grapefruit and Avocado Salad with Pine Nuts

1. In a large bowl, combine the mixed greens, grapefruit segments, diced avocado, and toasted pine nuts.

2. In a small bowl, whisk together the olive oil, white wine vinegar, honey, salt, and black pepper.

3. Drizzle the dressing over the salad and toss to coat evenly.

4. Serve immediately.

NUTRITION FACTS: Calories 240 | Total Fat 18g | Saturated Fat 2g | Cholesterol 0mg | Sodium 210mg | Total Carbohydrates 18g | Dietary Fiber 6g | Total Sugars 10g | Protein 4g

 **Preparation: 15 minutes**

 **Cook Time: 0 minutes**

 **Total Time: 15 minutes**

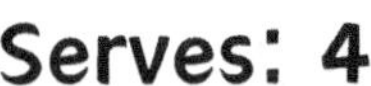 **Serves: 4**

- 4 cups cubed watermelon
- 1/2 cup crumbled feta cheese
- 1/4 cup chopped fresh mint
- 1/4 cup chopped walnuts, toasted
- 2 tablespoons olive oil
- 1 tablespoon balsamic vinegar
- 1 teaspoon honey
- 1/4 teaspoon salt
- 1/4 teaspoon black pepper

11. Watermelon and Mint Salad with Feta and Walnuts

1. In a large bowl, combine the cubed watermelon, crumbled feta cheese, chopped fresh mint, and toasted chopped walnuts.

2. In a small bowl, whisk together the olive oil, balsamic vinegar, honey, salt, and black pepper.

3. Drizzle the dressing over the salad and toss to coat evenly.

4. Serve immediately.

NUTRITION FACTS: Calories 190 | Total Fat 13g | Saturated Fat 3g | Cholesterol 15mg | Sodium 320mg | Total Carbohydrates 16g | Dietary Fiber 2g | Total Sugars 13g | Protein 5g

 **Preparation: 15 minutes**

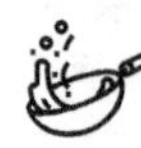 **Cook Time: 0 minutes**

 **Total Time: 15 minutes**

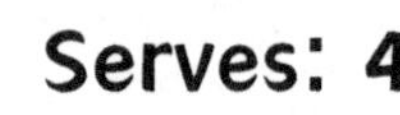 **Serves: 4**

- 4 cups baby arugula
- 2 ripe peaches, sliced
- 1/4 cup sliced almonds, toasted
- 2 tablespoons olive oil
- 1 tablespoon white balsamic vinegar
- 1 teaspoon honey
- 1/4 teaspoon salt
- 1/4 teaspoon black pepper

12. Peach and Arugula Salad with Almonds

1. In a large bowl, combine the baby arugula, sliced peaches, and toasted sliced almonds.

2. In a small bowl, whisk together the olive oil, white balsamic vinegar, honey, salt, and black pepper.

3. Drizzle the dressing over the salad and toss to coat evenly.

4. Serve immediately.

NUTRITION FACTS: Calories 160 | Total Fat 12g | Saturated Fat 2g | Cholesterol 0mg | Sodium 210mg | Total Carbohydrates 12g | Dietary Fiber 3g | Total Sugars 8g | Protein 4g

 **Preparation: 15 minutes**

 **Cook Time: 0 minutes**

 **Total Time: 15 minutes**

Serves: 4

- 5 cups baby greens (such as spinach, arugula, or mixed greens)
- 1 cup red grapes, halved
- 1/2 cup toasted walnuts, chopped
- 2 tablespoons olive oil
- 1 tablespoon white wine vinegar
- 1 teaspoon Dijon mustard
- 1 teaspoon honey
- 1/4 teaspoon salt
- 1/4 teaspoon black pepper

13. Grape and Walnut Salad with Baby Greens

1. In a large bowl, combine the baby greens, halved red grapes, and chopped toasted walnuts.

2. In a small bowl, whisk together the olive oil, white wine vinegar, Dijon mustard, honey, salt, and black pepper.

3. Drizzle the dressing over the salad and toss to coat evenly.

4. Serve immediately.

NUTRITION FACTS: Calories 190 | Total Fat 15g | Saturated Fat 2g | Cholesterol 0mg | Sodium 220mg | Total Carbohydrates 14g | Dietary Fiber 3g | Total Sugars 9g | Protein 4g

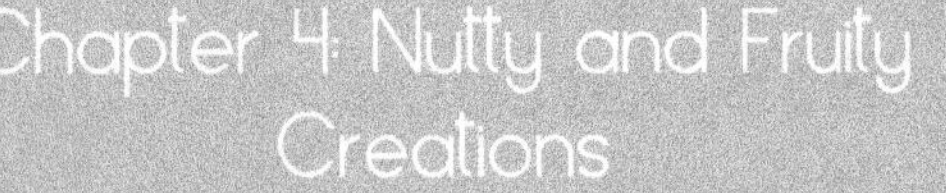

14. Cranberry and Pecan Salad with Mixed Greens

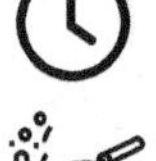 **Preparation: 15 minutes**

 **Cook Time: 0 minutes**

 **Total Time: 15 minutes**

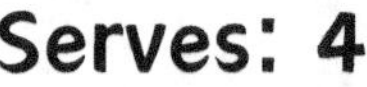 **Serves: 4**

- 6 cups mixed greens (such as spinach, arugula, and kale)
- 1/2 cup dried cranberries
- 1/2 cup toasted pecans, chopped
- 2 tablespoons olive oil
- 1 tablespoon balsamic vinegar
- 1 teaspoon Dijon mustard
- 1 teaspoon honey
- 1/4 teaspoon salt
- 1/4 teaspoon black pepper

1. In a large bowl, combine the mixed greens, dried cranberries, and chopped toasted pecans.

2. In a small bowl, whisk together the olive oil, balsamic vinegar, Dijon mustard, honey, salt, and black pepper.

3. Drizzle the dressing over the salad and toss to coat evenly.
4. Serve immediately.

NUTRITION FACTS: Calories 210 | Total Fat 15g | Saturated Fat 2g | Cholesterol 0mg | Sodium 240mg | Total Carbohydrates 18g | Dietary Fiber 4g | Total Sugars 12g | Protein 4g

🕐 **Preparation: 20 minutes**

Cook Time: 0 minutes

Total Time: 20 minutes

Serves: 4

- 4 cups mixed greens
- 1 ripe papaya, peeled, seeded, and cubed
- 1/2 cup chopped macadamia nuts, toasted
- 2 tablespoons olive oil
- 1 tablespoon lime juice
- 1 teaspoon honey
- 1/4 teaspoon salt
- 1/4 teaspoon black pepper

15. Papaya and Macadamia Nut Salad

1. In a large bowl, combine the mixed greens, cubed papaya, and toasted chopped macadamia nuts.
2. In a small bowl, whisk together the olive oil, lime juice, honey, salt, and black pepper.
3. Drizzle the dressing over the salad and toss to coat evenly.
4. Serve immediately.

NUTRITION FACTS: Calories 220 | Total Fat 17g | Saturated Fat 2g | Cholesterol 0mg | Sodium 210mg | Total Carbohydrates 15g | Dietary Fiber 4g | Total Sugars 10g | Protein 4g

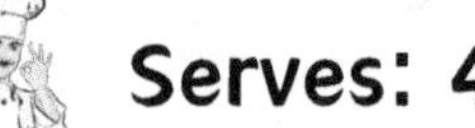

Preparation: 15 minutes

Cook Time: 0 minutes

Total Time: 15 minutes

Serves: 4

- 4 cups baby arugula
- 3 ripe plums, pitted and sliced
- 1/2 cup roasted and salted pistachios, chopped
- 2 tablespoons olive oil
- 1 tablespoon balsamic vinegar
- 1 teaspoon honey
- 1/4 teaspoon salt
- 1/4 teaspoon black pepper

16. Plum and Pistachio Salad with Arugula

1. In a large bowl, combine the baby arugula, sliced plums, and chopped roasted and salted pistachios.

2. In a small bowl, whisk together the olive oil, balsamic vinegar, honey, salt, and black pepper.

3. Drizzle the dressing over the salad and toss to coat evenly.

4. Serve immediately.

NUTRITION FACTS: Calories 180 | Total Fat 13g | Saturated Fat 2g | Cholesterol 0mg | Sodium 240mg | Total Carbohydrates 14g | Dietary Fiber 3g | Total Sugars 9g | Protein 5g

 **Preparation: 15 minutes**

 **Cook Time: 0 minutes**

 **Total Time: 15 minutes**

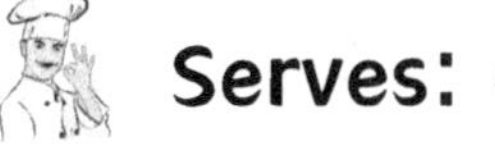 **Serves: 4**

- 5 cups baby spinach
- 2 kiwi fruits, peeled and sliced
- 1/2 cup roasted and salted cashews, chopped
- 2 tablespoons olive oil
- 1 tablespoon white wine vinegar
- 1 teaspoon Dijon mustard
- 1 teaspoon honey
- 1/4 teaspoon salt
- 1/4 teaspoon black pepper

17. Kiwi and Cashew Salad with Baby Spinach

1. In a large bowl, combine the baby spinach, sliced kiwi fruits, and chopped roasted and salted cashews.

2. In a small bowl, whisk together the olive oil, white wine vinegar, Dijon mustard, honey, salt, and black pepper.

3. Drizzle the dressing over the salad and toss to coat evenly.

4. Serve immediately.

NUTRITION FACTS: Calories 190 | Total Fat 14g | Saturated Fat 2g | Cholesterol 0mg | Sodium 240mg | Total Carbohydrates 14g | Dietary Fiber 4g | Total Sugars 8g | Protein 5g

18. Orange and Almond Salad with Mixed Greens

 **Preparation: 20 minutes**

 **Cook Time: 0 minutes**

Total Time: 20 minutes

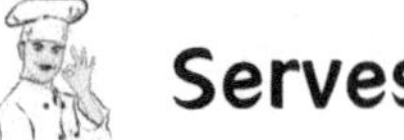 **Serves: 4**

- 6 cups mixed greens (such as spinach, arugula, and kale)
- 2 oranges, peeled and segmented
- 1/2 cup sliced almonds, toasted
- 2 tablespoons olive oil
- 1 tablespoon orange juice
- 1 tablespoon white wine vinegar
- 1 teaspoon honey
- 1/4 teaspoon salt
- 1/4 teaspoon black pepper

1. In a large bowl, combine the mixed greens, orange segments, and toasted sliced almonds.

2. In a small bowl, whisk together the olive oil, orange juice, white wine vinegar, honey, salt, and black pepper.

3. Drizzle the dressing over the salad and toss to coat evenly.

4. Serve immediately.

NUTRITION FACTS: Calories 210 | Total Fat 15g | Saturated Fat 2g | Cholesterol 0mg | Sodium 230mg | Total Carbohydrates 18g | Dietary Fiber 5g | Total Sugars 10g | Protein 5g

 **Preparation: 15 minutes**

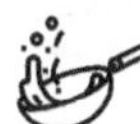 **Cook Time: 0 minutes**

 **Total Time: 15 minutes**

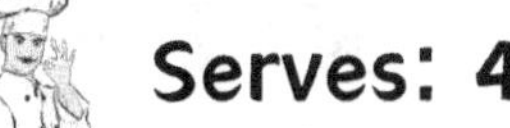 **Serves: 4**

- 5 cups baby kale
- 1 cup fresh blueberries
- 1/2 cup toasted pecans, chopped
- 2 tablespoons olive oil
- 1 tablespoon balsamic vinegar
- 1 teaspoon Dijon mustard
- 1 teaspoon honey
- 1/4 teaspoon salt
- 1/4 teaspoon black pepper

19. Blueberry and Pecan Salad with Baby Kale

1. In a large bowl, combine the baby kale, fresh blueberries, and chopped toasted pecans.

2. In a small bowl, whisk together the olive oil, balsamic vinegar, Dijon mustard, honey, salt, and black pepper.

3. Drizzle the dressing over the salad and toss to coat evenly.

4. Serve immediately.

NUTRITION FACTS: Calories 190 | Total Fat 14g | Saturated Fat 2g | Cholesterol 0mg | Sodium 240mg | Total Carbohydrates 15g | Dietary Fiber 4g | Total Sugars 9g | Protein 4g

 **Preparation: 15 minutes**

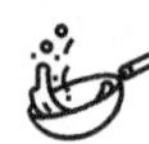 **Cook Time: 0 minutes**

 **Total Time: 15 minutes**

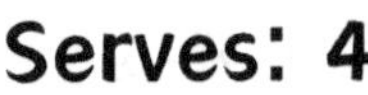 **Serves: 4**

- 6 cups mesclun mix (a blend of baby greens)
- 1 cup fresh blackberries
- 1/2 cup toasted walnuts, chopped
- 2 tablespoons olive oil
- 1 tablespoon balsamic vinegar
- 1 teaspoon Dijon mustard
- 1 teaspoon honey
- 1/4 teaspoon salt
- 1/4 teaspoon black pepper

20. Blackberry and Walnut Salad with Mesclun Mix

1. In a large bowl, combine the mesclun mix, fresh blackberries, and chopped toasted walnuts.

2. In a small bowl, whisk together the olive oil, balsamic vinegar, Dijon mustard, honey, salt, and black pepper.

3. Drizzle the dressing over the salad and toss to coat evenly.

4. Serve immediately.

NUTRITION FACTS: Calories 200 | Total Fat 15g | Saturated Fat 2g | Cholesterol 0mg | Sodium 230mg | Total Carbohydrates 15g | Dietary Fiber 5g | Total Sugars 8g | Protein 4g

1. Farro and Roasted Vegetable Salad with Lemon Vinaigrette

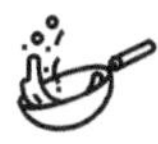 **Preparation: 20 minutes**

 **Cook Time: 30 minutes**

Total Time: 50 minutes

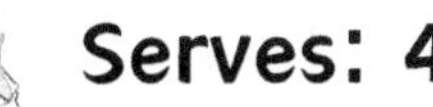 **Serves: 4**

- 1 cup uncooked farro
- 2 cups mixed roasted vegetables (such as bell peppers, zucchini, and onions)
- 1/2 cup crumbled feta cheese
- 2 tablespoons olive oil
- 2 tablespoons lemon juice
- 1 teaspoon Dijon mustard
- 1 teaspoon honey
- 1/4 teaspoon salt
- 1/4 teaspoon black pepper

1. Preheat the oven to 400°F.

2. Spread the mixed vegetables on a baking sheet and roast for 25-30 minutes, or until tender and lightly browned.

3. Meanwhile, cook the farro according to package instructions. Drain and let cool.

4. In a large bowl, combine the cooked farro, roasted vegetables, and crumbled feta cheese.

5. In a small bowl, whisk together the olive oil, lemon juice, Dijon mustard, honey, salt, and black pepper.

6. Drizzle the dressing over the salad and toss to coat evenly.

7. Serve immediately.

NUTRITION FACTS: Calories 320 | Total Fat 14g | Saturated Fat 4g | Cholesterol 20mg | Sodium 480mg | Total Carbohydrates 40g | Dietary Fiber 7g | Total Sugars 7g | Protein 10g

2. Quinoa and Black Bean Salad with Cilantro-Lime Dressing

 **Preparation: 20 minutes**

 **Cook Time: 15 minutes**

 **Total Time: 35 minutes**

Serves: 4

- 1 cup uncooked quinoa
- 1 (15 oz) can black beans, rinsed and drained
- 1 cup diced cucumber
- 1/2 cup diced red bell pepper
- 1/4 cup chopped fresh cilantro
- 2 tablespoons olive oil
- 2 tablespoons lime juice
- 1 teaspoon honey
- 1/4 teaspoon salt
- 1/4 teaspoon black pepper

1. Cook the quinoa according to package instructions. Fluff with a fork and let cool.

2. In a large bowl, combine the cooked quinoa, black beans, diced cucumber, diced red bell pepper, and chopped fresh cilantro.

3. In a small bowl, whisk together the olive oil, lime juice, honey, salt, and black pepper.

4. Drizzle the dressing over the salad and toss to coat evenly.

5. Serve immediately or refrigerate until ready to serve.

NUTRITION FACTS: Calories 280 | Total Fat 9g | Saturated Fat 1g | Cholesterol 0mg | Sodium 420mg | Total Carbohydrates 40g | Dietary Fiber 9g | Total Sugars 5g | Protein 10g

🕐 **Preparation: 15 minutes**

Cook Time: 45 minutes

Total Time: 1 hour

Serves: 4

- 1 cup uncooked wild rice
- 1/2 cup dried cranberries
- 1/2 cup chopped pecans, toasted
- 2 tablespoons olive oil
- 2 tablespoons apple cider vinegar
- 1 teaspoon Dijon mustard
- 1 teaspoon honey
- 1/4 teaspoon salt
- 1/4 teaspoon black pepper

3. Wild Rice and Cranberry Salad with Pecans

1. Cook the wild rice according to package instructions. Drain and let cool.

2. In a large bowl, combine the cooked wild rice, dried cranberries, and toasted chopped pecans.

3. In a small bowl, whisk together the olive oil, apple cider vinegar, Dijon mustard, honey, salt, and black pepper.

4. Drizzle the dressing over the salad and toss to coat evenly.

5. Serve immediately or refrigerate until ready to serve.

NUTRITION FACTS: Calories 290 | Total Fat 14g | Saturated Fat 2g | Cholesterol 0mg | Sodium 240mg | Total Carbohydrates 37g | Dietary Fiber 5g | Total Sugars 12g | Protein 6g

4. Chickpea and Cucumber Salad with Dill

🕐 **Preparation: 15 minutes**

🥄 **Cook Time: 0 minutes**

✓ **Total Time: 15 minutes**

👨‍🍳 **Serves: 4**

- 1 (15 oz) can chickpeas, rinsed and drained
- 1 cup diced cucumber
- 1/4 cup chopped fresh dill
- 2 tablespoons olive oil
- 2 tablespoons lemon juice
- 1 teaspoon Dijon mustard
- 1/4 teaspoon salt
- 1/4 teaspoon black pepper

1. In a large bowl, combine the rinsed and drained chickpeas, diced cucumber, and chopped fresh dill.

2. In a small bowl, whisk together the olive oil, lemon juice, Dijon mustard, salt, and black pepper.

3. Drizzle the dressing over the salad and toss to coat evenly.

4. Serve immediately or refrigerate until ready to serve.

NUTRITION FACTS: Calories 180 | Total Fat 9g | Saturated Fat 1g | Cholesterol 0mg | Sodium 360mg | Total Carbohydrates 20g | Dietary Fiber 5g | Total Sugars 3g | Protein 6g

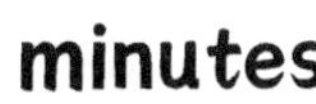

5. Lentil and Roasted Beet Salad with Feta

🕐 **Preparation: 20 minutes**

Cook Time: 45 minutes

Total Time: 1 hour 5 minutes

Serves: 4

- 1 cup uncooked lentils, rinsed
- 3 medium beets, peeled and cut into 1-inch cubes
- 2 tablespoons olive oil, divided
- 1/4 cup crumbled feta cheese
- 2 tablespoons balsamic vinegar
- 1 teaspoon Dijon mustard
- 1 teaspoon honey
- 1/4 teaspoon salt
- 1/4 teaspoon black pepper

1. Preheat the oven to 400°F.

2. Toss the cubed beets with 1 tablespoon of olive oil and spread them on a baking sheet. Roast for 35-45 minutes, or until tender and lightly caramelized.

3. Meanwhile, cook the lentils according to package instructions. Drain and let cool.

4. In a large bowl, combine the cooked lentils, roasted beets, and crumbled feta cheese.

5. In a small bowl, whisk together the remaining 1 tablespoon of olive oil, balsamic vinegar, Dijon mustard, honey, salt, and black pepper.

6. Drizzle the dressing over the salad and toss to coat evenly.

7. Serve immediately or refrigerate until ready to serve.

NUTRITION FACTS: Calories 260 | Total Fat 10g | Saturated Fat 3g | Cholesterol 15mg | Sodium 420mg | Total Carbohydrates 32g | Dietary Fiber 10g | Total Sugars 10g | Protein 12g

6. Barley and Mushroom Salad with Thyme

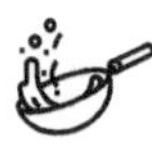 **Preparation: 15 minutes**

 **Cook Time: 30 minutes**

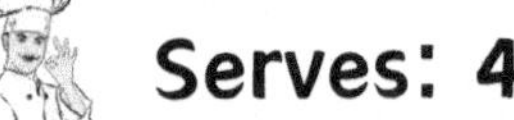 **Total Time: 45 minutes**

Serves: 4

- 1 cup uncooked pearl barley
- 8 oz sliced mushrooms
- 2 tablespoons olive oil
- 1 tablespoon balsamic vinegar
- 1 tablespoon chopped fresh thyme
- 1 teaspoon Dijon mustard
- 1/4 teaspoon salt
- 1/4 teaspoon black pepper

1. Cook the barley according to package instructions. Drain and let cool.

2. In a large skillet, heat 1 tablespoon of olive oil over medium-high heat. Add the sliced mushrooms and sauté for 5-7 minutes, or until they are tender and lightly browned.

3. In a large bowl, combine the cooked barley, sautéed mushrooms, and chopped fresh thyme.

4. In a small bowl, whisk together the remaining 1 tablespoon of olive oil, balsamic vinegar, Dijon mustard, salt, and black pepper.

5. Drizzle the dressing over the salad and toss to coat evenly.

6. Serve immediately or refrigerate until ready to serve.

NUTRITION FACTS: Calories 220 | Total Fat 8g | Saturated Fat 1g | Cholesterol 0mg | Sodium 320mg | Total Carbohydrates 32g | Dietary Fiber 6g | Total Sugars 2g | Protein 6g

7. Bulgar Wheat and Parsley Salad with Lemon

 **Preparation: 15 minutes**

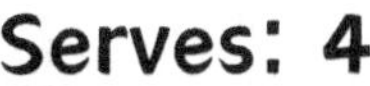 **Cook Time: 15 minutes**

Total Time: 30 minutes

Serves: 4

- 1 cup uncooked bulgar wheat
- 1 cup chopped fresh parsley
- 2 tablespoons olive oil
- 2 tablespoons lemon juice
- 1 teaspoon lemon zest
- 1 teaspoon honey
- 1/4 teaspoon salt
- 1/4 teaspoon black pepper

1. Cook the bulgar wheat according to package instructions. Drain and let cool.

2. In a large bowl, combine the cooked bulgar wheat and chopped fresh parsley.

3. In a small bowl, whisk together the olive oil, lemon juice, lemon zest, honey, salt, and black pepper.

4. Drizzle the dressing over the salad and toss to coat evenly.

5. Serve immediately or refrigerate until ready to serve.

NUTRITION FACTS: Calories 190 | Total Fat 8g | Saturated Fat 1g | Cholesterol 0mg | Sodium 240mg | Total Carbohydrates 26g | Dietary Fiber 5g | Total Sugars 4g | Protein 5g

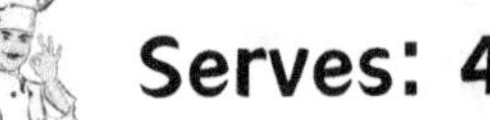

⏰ **Preparation: 20 minutes**

🥣 **Cook Time: 20 minutes**

✅ **Total Time: 40 minutes**

👨‍🍳 **Serves: 4**

- 1 cup uncooked millet
- 1 cup diced bell peppers (mix of red, yellow, and orange)
- 1 cup diced zucchini
- 1/2 cup diced red onion
- 2 tablespoons olive oil
- 2 tablespoons apple cider vinegar
- 1 teaspoon Dijon mustard
- 1 teaspoon honey
- 1/4 teaspoon salt
- 1/4 teaspoon black pepper

8. Millet and Mixed Vegetable Salad

1. Cook the millet according to package instructions. Fluff with a fork and let cool.

2. In a large bowl, combine the cooked millet, diced bell peppers, diced zucchini, and diced red onion.

3. In a small bowl, whisk together the olive oil, apple cider vinegar, Dijon mustard, honey, salt, and black pepper.

4. Drizzle the dressing over the salad and toss to coat evenly.

5. Serve immediately or refrigerate until ready to serve.

NUTRITION FACTS: Calories 240 | Total Fat 9g | Saturated Fat 1g | Cholesterol 0mg | Sodium 320mg | Total Carbohydrates 35g | Dietary Fiber 5g | Total Sugars 7g | Protein 6g

9. Brown Rice and Edamame Salad with Ginger Dressing

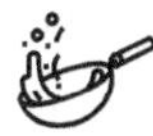 **Preparation: 20 minutes**

 **Cook Time: 30 minutes**

Total Time: 50 minutes

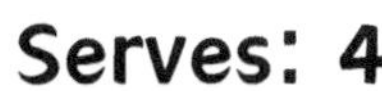 **Serves: 4**

- 1 cup uncooked brown rice
- 1 cup shelled edamame
- 1/2 cup diced cucumber
- 1/4 cup chopped green onions
- 2 tablespoons olive oil
- 1 tablespoon rice vinegar
- 1 teaspoon grated fresh ginger
- 1 teaspoon honey
- 1/4 teaspoon salt
- 1/4 teaspoon black pepper

1. Cook the brown rice according to package instructions. Fluff with a fork and let cool.

2. In a large bowl, combine the cooked brown rice, shelled edamame, diced cucumber, and chopped green onions.

3. In a small bowl, whisk together the olive oil, rice vinegar, grated fresh ginger, honey, salt, and black pepper.

4. Drizzle the dressing over the salad and toss to coat evenly.

5. Serve immediately or refrigerate until ready to serve.

NUTRITION FACTS: Calories 260 | Total Fat 9g | Saturated Fat 1g | Cholesterol 0mg | Sodium 260mg | Total Carbohydrates 35g | Dietary Fiber 5g | Total Sugars 4g | Protein 10g

10. Quinoa, Spinach, and Avocado Salad

 **Preparation: 15 minutes**

 **Cook Time: 15 minutes**

 **Total Time: 30 minutes**

Serves: 4

- 1 cup uncooked quinoa
- 4 cups baby spinach
- 1 avocado, diced
- 2 tablespoons olive oil
- 2 tablespoons lemon juice
- 1 teaspoon Dijon mustard
- 1 teaspoon honey
- 1/4 teaspoon salt
- 1/4 teaspoon black pepper

1. Cook the quinoa according to package instructions. Fluff with a fork and let cool.

2. In a large bowl, combine the cooked quinoa, baby spinach, and diced avocado.

3. In a small bowl, whisk together the olive oil, lemon juice, Dijon mustard, honey, salt, and black pepper.

4. Drizzle the dressing over the salad and toss to coat evenly.

5. Serve immediately or refrigerate until ready to serve.

NUTRITION FACTS: Calories 290 | Total Fat 15g | Saturated Fat 2g | Cholesterol 0mg | Sodium 320mg | Total Carbohydrates 32g | Dietary Fiber 8g | Total Sugars 4g | Protein 8g

11. Lentil and Carrot Salad with Tahini Dressing

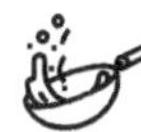 **Preparation: 20 minutes**

 **Cook Time: 20 minutes**

Total Time: 40 minutes

Serves: 4

- 1 cup uncooked lentils, rinsed
- 2 cups diced carrots
- 1/4 cup chopped fresh parsley
- 2 tablespoons tahini
- 2 tablespoons lemon juice
- 1 tablespoon water
- 1 teaspoon honey
- 1/4 teaspoon ground cumin
- 1/4 teaspoon salt
- 1/4 teaspoon black pepper

1. Cook the lentils according to package instructions. Drain and let cool.

2. In a large bowl, combine the cooked lentils, diced carrots, and chopped fresh parsley.

3. In a small bowl, whisk together the tahini, lemon juice, water, honey, ground cumin, salt, and black pepper.

4. Drizzle the tahini dressing over the salad and toss to coat evenly.

5. Serve immediately or refrigerate until ready to serve.

NUTRITION FACTS: Calories 260 | Total Fat 9g | Saturated Fat 1g | Cholesterol 0mg | Sodium 320mg | Total Carbohydrates 34g | Dietary Fiber 12g | Total Sugars 7g | Protein 13g

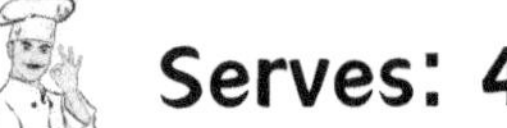

Preparation: 15 minutes

Cook Time: 20 minutes

Total Time: 35 minutes

Serves: 4

- 1 cup uncooked farro
- 4 cups baby arugula
- 1/2 cup pomegranate seeds
- 2 tablespoons olive oil
- 2 tablespoons balsamic vinegar
- 1 teaspoon Dijon mustard
- 1 teaspoon honey
- 1/4 teaspoon salt
- 1/4 teaspoon black pepper

12. Farro and Arugula Salad with Pomegranate Seeds

1. Cook the farro according to package instructions. Drain and let cool.

2. In a large bowl, combine the cooked farro, baby arugula, and pomegranate seeds.

3. In a small bowl, whisk together the olive oil, balsamic vinegar, Dijon mustard, honey, salt, and black pepper.

4. Drizzle the dressing over the salad and toss to coat evenly.

5. Serve immediately or refrigerate until ready to serve.

NUTRITION FACTS: Calories 270 | Total Fat 10g | Saturated Fat 1g | Cholesterol 0mg | Sodium 320mg | Total Carbohydrates 38g | Dietary Fiber 7g | Total Sugars 8g | Protein 8g

13. Barley and Beet Salad with Goat Cheese

 **Preparation: 20 minutes**

 **Cook Time: 40 minutes**

Total Time: 1 hour

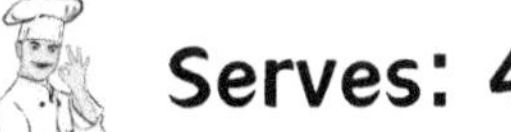 **Serves: 4**

- 1 cup uncooked pearl barley
- 3 medium beets, peeled and diced
- 2 tablespoons olive oil
- 2 tablespoons red wine vinegar
- 1 teaspoon Dijon mustard
- 1 teaspoon honey
- 1/4 teaspoon salt
- 1/4 teaspoon black pepper
- 1/2 cup crumbled goat cheese

1. Cook the barley according to package instructions. Drain and let cool.

2. Preheat the oven to 400°F. Toss the diced beets with 1 tablespoon of olive oil and spread them on a baking sheet. Roast for 30-40 minutes, or until tender and lightly caramelized.

3. In a large bowl, combine the cooked barley, roasted beets, and crumbled goat cheese.

4. In a small bowl, whisk together the remaining 1 tablespoon of olive oil, red wine vinegar, Dijon mustard, honey, salt, and black pepper.

5. Drizzle the dressing over the salad and toss to coat evenly.

6. Serve immediately or refrigerate until ready to serve.

NUTRITION FACTS: Calories 280 | Total Fat 12g | Saturated Fat 4g | Cholesterol 15mg | Sodium 420mg | Total Carbohydrates 34g | Dietary Fiber 6g | Total Sugars 8g | Protein 9g

14. Chickpea and Red Pepper Salad with Lemon Vinaigrette

 **Preparation: 15 minutes**

 **Cook Time: 0 minutes**

 **Total Time: 15 minutes**

Serves: 4

- 1 (15 oz) can chickpeas, rinsed and drained
- 1 red bell pepper, diced
- 1/4 cup chopped fresh parsley
- 2 tablespoons olive oil
- 2 tablespoons lemon juice
- 1 teaspoon Dijon mustard
- 1 teaspoon honey
- 1/4 teaspoon salt
- 1/4 teaspoon black pepper

1. In a large bowl, combine the rinsed and drained chickpeas, diced red bell pepper, and chopped fresh parsley.

2. In a small bowl, whisk together the olive oil, lemon juice, Dijon mustard, honey, salt, and black pepper.

3. Drizzle the lemon vinaigrette over the chickpea and red pepper salad and toss to coat evenly.

4. Serve immediately or refrigerate until ready to serve.

NUTRITION FACTS: Calories 200 | Total Fat 9g | Saturated Fat 1g | Cholesterol 0mg | Sodium 360mg | Total Carbohydrates 24g | Dietary Fiber 6g | Total Sugars 5g | Protein 7g

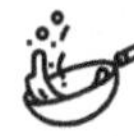

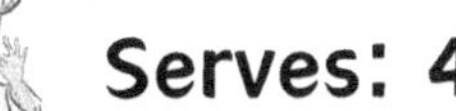

Preparation: 15 minutes

Cook Time: 0 minutes

Total Time: 15 minutes

Serves: 4

- 1 (15 oz) can black beans, rinsed and drained
- 1 cup frozen corn, thawed
- 1/2 cup diced red onion
- 1/4 cup chopped fresh cilantro
- 2 tablespoons olive oil
- 2 tablespoons lime juice
- 1 teaspoon honey
- 1/4 teaspoon ground cumin
- 1/4 teaspoon salt
- 1/4 teaspoon black pepper

15. Black Bean and Corn Salad with Lime-Cilantro Dressing

1. In a large bowl, combine the rinsed and drained black beans, thawed corn, diced red onion, and chopped fresh cilantro.

2. In a small bowl, whisk together the olive oil, lime juice, honey, ground cumin, salt, and black pepper.

3. Drizzle the lime-cilantro dressing over the black bean and corn salad and toss to coat evenly.

4. Serve immediately or refrigerate until ready to serve.

NUTRITION FACTS: Calories 210 | Total Fat 7g | Saturated Fat 1g | Cholesterol 0mg | Sodium 420mg | Total Carbohydrates 30g | Dietary Fiber 8g | Total Sugars 5g | Protein 8g

16. Wild Rice and Kale Salad with Orange Dressing

 **Preparation: 20 minutes**

 **Cook Time: 45 minutes**

Total Time:55 minutes

Serves: 4

- 1 cup uncooked wild rice
- 4 cups chopped kale
- 1/2 cup diced orange segments
- 2 tablespoons olive oil
- 2 tablespoons orange juice
- 1 tablespoon apple cider vinegar
- 1 teaspoon Dijon mustard
- 1 teaspoon honey
- 1/4 teaspoon salt
- 1/4 teaspoon black pepper

1. Cook the wild rice according to package instructions. Drain and let cool.

2. In a large bowl, combine the cooked wild rice, chopped kale, and diced orange segments.

3. In a small bowl, whisk together the olive oil, orange juice, apple cider vinegar, Dijon mustard, honey, salt, and black pepper.

4. Drizzle the orange dressing over the salad and toss to coat evenly.

5. Serve immediately or refrigerate until ready to serve.

NUTRITION FACTS: Calories 260 | Total Fat 8g | Saturated Fat 1g | Cholesterol 0mg | Sodium 320mg | Total Carbohydrates 40g | Dietary Fiber 5g | Total Sugars 9g | Protein 7g

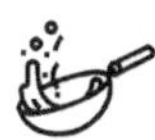

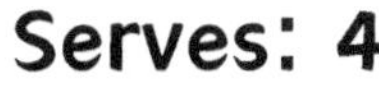

Preparation: 20 minutes

Cook Time: 30 minutes

Total Time: 50 minutes

Serves: 4

- 1 cup uncooked quinoa
- 2 cups diced sweet potatoes
- 2 tablespoons olive oil, divided
- 2 tablespoons tahini
- 2 tablespoons lemon juice
- 1 tablespoon water
- 1 teaspoon honey
- 1/4 teaspoon ground cumin
- 1/4 teaspoon salt
- 1/4 teaspoon black pepper
- 2 tablespoons chopped fresh parsley

17. Quinoa and Sweet Potato Salad with Tahini Dressing

1. Cook the quinoa according to package instructions. Fluff with a fork and let cool.

2. Preheat the oven to 400°F. Toss the diced sweet potatoes with 1 tablespoon of olive oil and spread them on a baking sheet. Roast for 25-30 minutes, or until tender and lightly browned.

3. In a small bowl, whisk together the remaining 1 tablespoon of olive oil, tahini, lemon juice, water, honey, ground cumin, salt, and black pepper.

4. In a large bowl, combine the cooked quinoa, roasted sweet potatoes, and chopped fresh parsley.

5. Drizzle the tahini dressing over the salad and toss to coat evenly.

6. Serve immediately or refrigerate until ready to serve.

NUTRITION FACTS: Calories 320 | Total Fat 12g | Saturated Fat 2g | Cholesterol 0mg | Sodium 320mg | Total Carbohydrates 44g | Dietary Fiber 6g | Total Sugars 8g | Protein 9g

18. Lentil and Spinach Salad with Walnut Dressing

 **Preparation: 20 minutes**

 **Cook Time: 20 minutes**

Total Time: 40 minutes

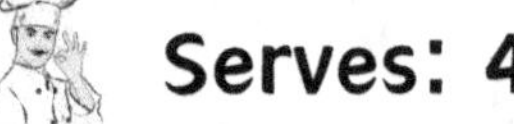 **Serves: 4**

- 1 cup uncooked lentils, rinsed
- 4 cups baby spinach
- 1/4 cup chopped walnuts, toasted
- 2 tablespoons olive oil
- 2 tablespoons walnut oil
- 2 tablespoons balsamic vinegar
- 1 teaspoon Dijon mustard
- 1 teaspoon honey
- 1/4 teaspoon salt
- 1/4 teaspoon black pepper

1. Cook the lentils according to package instructions. Drain and let cool.

2. In a large bowl, combine the cooked lentils, baby spinach, and toasted chopped walnuts.

3. In a small bowl, whisk together the olive oil, walnut oil, balsamic vinegar, Dijon mustard, honey, salt, and black pepper.

4. Drizzle the walnut dressing over the salad and toss to coat evenly.

5. Serve immediately or refrigerate until ready to serve.

NUTRITION FACTS: Calories 280 | Total Fat 15g | Saturated Fat 2g | Cholesterol 0mg | Sodium 320mg | Total Carbohydrates 25g | Dietary Fiber 9g | Total Sugars 5g | Protein 12g

🕐 **Preparation: 20 minutes**

Cook Time: 40 minutes

Total Time: 1 hour

Serves: 4

- 1 cup uncooked freekeh
- 2 cups mixed roasted vegetables (such as zucchini, bell peppers, and onions)
- 2 tablespoons olive oil
- 2 tablespoons balsamic vinegar
- 1 teaspoon Dijon mustard
- 1 teaspoon honey
- 1/4 teaspoon salt
- 1/4 teaspoon black pepper
- 2 tablespoons chopped fresh parsley

19. Freekeh and Roasted Vegetable Salad

1. Cook the freekeh according to package instructions. Drain and let cool.

2. Preheat the oven to 400°F. Toss the mixed vegetables with 1 tablespoon of olive oil and spread them on a baking sheet. Roast for 30-40 minutes, or until tender and lightly caramelized.

3. In a large bowl, combine the cooked freekeh, roasted vegetables, and chopped fresh parsley.

4. In a small bowl, whisk together the remaining 1 tablespoon of olive oil, balsamic vinegar, Dijon mustard, honey, salt, and black pepper.

5. Drizzle the dressing over the salad and toss to coat evenly.

6. Serve immediately or refrigerate until ready to serve.

NUTRITION FACTS: Calories 280 | Total Fat 10g | Saturated Fat 1g | Cholesterol 0mg | Sodium 420mg | Total Carbohydrates 40g | Dietary Fiber 8g | Total Sugars 7g | Protein 8g

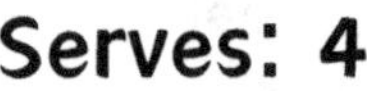

Preparation: 20 minutes

Cook Time: 20 minutes

Total Time: 40 minutes

Serves: 4

- 1 cup uncooked farro
- 2 cups halved cherry tomatoes
- 1/4 cup basil pesto
- 2 tablespoons olive oil
- 1 tablespoon balsamic vinegar
- 1/4 teaspoon salt
- 1/4 teaspoon black pepper
- 2 tablespoons toasted pine nuts

20. Farro and Cherry Tomato Salad with Basil Pesto

1. Cook the farro according to package instructions. Drain and let cool.

2. In a large bowl, combine the cooked farro, halved cherry tomatoes, and basil pesto.

3. In a small bowl, whisk together the olive oil, balsamic vinegar, salt, and black pepper.

4. Drizzle the dressing over the salad and toss to coat evenly.

5. Sprinkle the toasted pine nuts over the top.

6. Serve immediately or refrigerate until ready to serve.

NUTRITION FACTS: Calories 320 | Total Fat 16g | Saturated Fat 3g | Cholesterol 0mg | Sodium 360mg | Total Carbohydrates 38g | Dietary Fiber 6g | Total Sugars 5g | Protein 9g

Creating a one-week anti-inflammatory diet plan involves focusing on whole foods, healthy fats, lean proteins, and plenty of fruits and vegetables. Here's a plan that includes breakfast, lunch, dinner, and snacks for each day:

Day 1
- Breakfast: Overnight oats with blueberries, chia seeds, and almond milk.
- Lunch: Quinoa salad with chickpeas, cucumber, tomatoes, and olive oil dressing.
- Dinner: Baked salmon with roasted sweet potatoes and steamed broccoli.
- Snacks: Carrot sticks with hummus, apple slices with almond butter.

Day 2
- Breakfast: Smoothie with spinach, banana, mixed berries, and flaxseeds.
- Lunch: Lentil soup with a side of mixed green salad.
- Dinner: Grilled chicken breast with quinoa and sautéed spinach.
- Snacks: Mixed nuts, orange slices.

Day 3
- Breakfast: Greek yogurt with honey, walnuts, and fresh strawberries.
- Lunch: Whole grain wrap with avocado, turkey, spinach, and tomatoes.
- Dinner: Stir-fried tofu with bell peppers, broccoli, and brown rice.
- Snacks: Celery sticks with guacamole, pear slices.

Day 4
- Breakfast: Chia pudding with mango and coconut flakes.
- Lunch: Mixed greens with grilled shrimp, avocado, and lemon vinaigrette.
- Dinner: Turkey meatballs with zucchini noodles and marinara sauce.
- Snacks: Almonds, blueberries.

Day 5
- Breakfast: Scrambled eggs with spinach, tomatoes, and avocado.
- Lunch: Farro salad with roasted vegetables and a balsamic glaze.
- Dinner: Baked cod with quinoa and a side of roasted Brussels sprouts.
- Snacks: Sliced cucumber with hummus, banana.

Day 6
- Breakfast: Smoothie bowl with acai, banana, granola, and chia seeds.
- Lunch: Chickpea and avocado salad with a side of mixed greens.
- Dinner: Grilled chicken thighs with roasted carrots and steamed green beans.
- Snacks: Apple slices with peanut butter, cherry tomatoes.

Day 7
- Breakfast: Oatmeal with almond butter, sliced banana, and cinnamon.
- Lunch: Spinach and quinoa salad with grilled tofu and tahini dressing.
- Dinner: Stuffed bell peppers with brown rice, black beans, and corn.
- Snacks: Trail mix, watermelon slices.

Here are some tips to help you follow an anti-inflammatory diet effectively:

1. Focus on Whole Foods
- Prioritize whole, unprocessed foods like fruits, vegetables, whole grains, nuts, seeds, and lean proteins.
- Avoid processed foods, refined sugars, and artificial additives.

2. Incorporate Healthy Fats
- Include sources of healthy fats such as olive oil, avocados, nuts, and seeds.
- Use fatty fish like salmon, mackerel, and sardines which are high in omega-3 fatty acids.

3. Eat a Rainbow of Fruits and Vegetables
- Aim for a variety of colorful fruits and vegetables to ensure a wide range of nutrients.
- Berries, leafy greens, tomatoes, peppers, and citrus fruits are particularly beneficial.

4. Choose Whole Grains
- Opt for whole grains like quinoa, brown rice, oats, barley, and whole wheat over refined grains.
- These provide fiber and essential nutrients that help reduce inflammation.

5. Stay Hydrated
- Drink plenty of water throughout the day.
- Herbal teas and water infused with fruits and herbs are also good options.

6. Limit Red Meat and Processed Meats
- Choose lean proteins such as poultry, fish, tofu, and legumes.
- If consuming red meat, opt for lean cuts and limit intake.

7. Include Anti-inflammatory Spices and Herbs
- Incorporate spices like turmeric, ginger, garlic, and cinnamon into your meals.
- These have natural anti-inflammatory properties.

8. Reduce Sugar and Salt Intake
- Minimize consumption of sugary drinks, sweets, and snacks.
- Use herbs, spices, and natural seasonings instead of salt to flavor your food.

9. Consider Probiotics and Prebiotics
- Include probiotic-rich foods like yogurt, kefir, sauerkraut, and kimchi.
- Prebiotic foods such as garlic, onions, and bananas support gut health.

10. Practice Mindful Eating
- Eat slowly and savor your food to promote better digestion and satisfaction.
- Pay attention to portion sizes and avoid overeating.

By incorporating these tips into your daily routine, you can effectively manage inflammation and support your overall health and well-being.

As we reach the conclusion of the *Anti-Inflammatory Salad Cookbook*, it's clear that the path to better health can be both delicious and enjoyable. By integrating these anti-inflammatory salads into your daily routine, you are not just adopting a healthier diet, but also taking proactive steps to manage inflammation and enhance your overall well-being.

Combining Salads for a Balanced Anti-Inflammatory Diet

A balanced diet is crucial for maintaining good health, and salads offer an excellent way to achieve this balance. The recipes in this cookbook are designed to provide a variety of nutrients from different food groups, ensuring that your body gets what it needs to function optimally. By combining leafy greens, cruciferous vegetables, lean proteins, healthy fats, and whole grains, these salads provide a comprehensive approach to fighting inflammation. Remember to mix and match these salads throughout the week to keep your meals interesting and nutritionally diverse.

Customizing Your Salads for Personal Taste and Health Needs

One of the greatest benefits of salads is their versatility. Each recipe in this book can be customized to suit your personal taste preferences and dietary requirements. If you're vegan or vegetarian, many of the salads can be easily adapted by swapping out animal proteins for plant-based alternatives. If you have specific health concerns, such as diabetes or heart disease, you can modify the ingredients and dressings to better suit your needs. Don't hesitate to experiment with different combinations and flavors to find what works best for you.

Embracing a Healthier Lifestyle

Incorporating anti-inflammatory salads into your diet is just one aspect of a healthier lifestyle. Regular physical activity, adequate sleep, and stress management are also critical components of overall well-being. As you continue to enjoy these salads, consider how other lifestyle changes can complement your dietary efforts. For instance, practicing mindfulness while eating, staying hydrated, and avoiding processed foods can further enhance the benefits of your anti-inflammatory diet.

Additional Resources and References for Anti-Inflammatory Diets

For those interested in diving deeper into the science of inflammation and diet, there are numerous resources available. Books, research articles, and reputable websites can provide further insights and tips on managing inflammation through food and lifestyle choices.

Thank you for embarking on this culinary adventure with us. We hope that these recipes inspire you to embrace the anti-inflammatory lifestyle and that they become a cherished part of your culinary repertoire. Here's to your health and happiness—one delicious salad at a time.